Myofascial Release

Hands-On Guides for Therapists

SECOND EDITION

Ruth Duncan, BSc (Hons), MSMTO

Myofascial Release UK

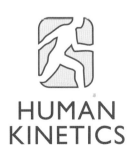

HUMAN KINETICS

Library of Congress Cataloging-in-Publication Data

Names: Duncan, Ruth A., 1968-
Title: Myofascial release / Ruth Duncan.
Other titles: Hands-on guides for therapists.
Description: Second edition. | Champaign : Human Kinetics, Inc., [2022] | Series: Hands-on guides for therapists | Includes bibliographical references and index.
Identifiers: LCCN 2021007255 (print) | LCCN 2021007256 (ebook) | ISBN 9781718200715 (paperback) | ISBN 9781718200722 (epub) | ISBN 9781718200739 (pdf)
Subjects: MESH: Manipulation, Orthopedic—methods | Fascia—physiology
Classification: LCC RM721 (print) | LCC RM721 (ebook) | NLM WB 535 | DDC 615.8/22—dc23
LC record available at https://lccn.loc.gov/2021007255
LC ebook record available at https://lccn.loc.gov/2021007256

ISBN: 978-1-7182-0071-5 (print)

Acquisitions Editor: Jolynn Gower; **Managing Editor:** Anna Lan Seaman; **Copyeditor:** Marissa Wold Uhrina; **Permissions Manager:** Dalene Reeder; **Senior Graphic Designer:** Nancy Rasmus; **Cover Designer:** Keri Evans; **Cover Design Specialist:** Susan Rothermel Allen; **Photograph (cover):** Ruth Duncan; **Photographs (interior):** Helen & David Roscoe-Rutter; © Human Kinetics, unless otherwise noted; **Photo Asset Manager:** Laura Fitch; **Photo Production Specialist:** Amy M. Rose; **Photo Production Manager:** Jason Allen; **Senior Art Manager:** Kelly Hendren; **Illustrations:** © Human Kinetics; **Production:** Westchester Publishing Services; **Printer:** Versa Press

Printed in the United States of America   10   9   8   7   6   5   4   3   2   1

The paper in this book is certified under a sustainable forestry program.

Human Kinetics
1607 N. Market Street
Champaign, IL 61820
USA

United States and International
Website: **US.HumanKinetics.com**
Email: info@hkusa.com
Phone: 1-800-747-4457

Canada
Website: **Canada.HumanKinetics.com**
Email: info@hkcanada.com

E8198

Tell us what you think!
Human Kinetics would love to hear what we can do to improve the customer experience. Use this QR code to take our brief survey.

Contents

Series Preface   vii • Preface   ix • Acknowledgements   xiii

PART I   Getting Started With Myofascial Release

1   Introduction to Myofascial Release   3

Elements of Fascia   4
Conditions That Affect Fascia   12
Myofascial Release Concepts   14
MFR Versus Other Massage Modalities   21
Benefits of MFR   21
MFR Treatment Sessions   22
Closing Remarks   23
Quick Questions   23

2   Initial Assessment   25

Client Consultation   26
Medical History   33
Physical Assessment   36
Postural Assessments   44
Closing Remarks   47
Quick Questions   47

3   Preparation and Communication   49

Contraindications   49
Equipment and Room Preparation   52
Correct Body Mechanics   54
Mental Preparation   56
Therapist and Client Communication   57
Effects of and Responses to MFR   58
Closing Remarks   62
Quick Questions   62

PART II   MFR Applications

4 Palpatory and Physical Assessments   65

Palpatory Assessment   65
Tissue Mobility and Glide   74
Traction and Compression   78
Skin Rolling   81
Rebounding   83
Closing Remarks   86
Quick Questions   86

5 MFR Technique Approaches   87

How to Apply Every MFR Technique   87
Cross-Hand Releases   92
Longitudinal Plane Releases   94
Compression Releases   96
Transverse Plane Releases   97
Scar Tissue and Adhesion Management   98
Myofascial Mobilisations   98
Combining Techniques   99
Closing Remarks   100
Quick Questions   100

PART III   Applying MFR Techniques

6 Cross-Hand Release Approaches   103

Leg Techniques   104
Arm Techniques   112
Torso Techniques   113
Head and Neck Techniques   122
Closing Remarks   123
Quick Questions   123

7 Longitudinal Plane Releases   125

Supine Pulls   127
Prone Pulls   131
Bilateral Pulls   133
Oppositional and Side-Lying Pulls   135
Closing Remarks   138
Quick Questions   138

8 Compression Releases   139

Soft Tissue Compression Techniques   141
Joint Compression Techniques   146

Closing Remarks   148
Quick Questions   148

9 Transverse Plane Releases   149

Pelvic Floor Techniques   150
Respiratory Diaphragm Techniques   151
Thoracic Inlet Techniques   152
Transverse Plane Techniques at Joints   154
Closing Remarks   155
Quick Questions   155

10 Scar Tissue and Adhesion Management   157

Scar Tissue Techniques   159
Stacking the Position of Ease Techniques   163
Direct Scar Tissue Release Techniques   169
Closing Remarks   171
Quick Questions   171

11 Myofascial Mobilisations   173

Applying Myofascial Mobilisation   175
Myofascial Mobilisation Techniques   179
Closing Remarks   196
Quick Questions   196

PART IV MFR Programmes and Management

12 Combined Techniques and Taking MFR Further   199

Myofascial Position of Ease Techniques   200
Combining Techniques   203
Closing Remarks   208
Quick Questions   208

13 MFR Treatment Approaches   209

Individual Treatment Approaches   210
Intensive Treatment Approaches   211
Multi-Therapist Treatment Approaches   212
Home Programmes   213
Closing Remarks   222
Quick Questions   222

Answers to Quick Questions   223 • References   227 •
Photo Index   229 • About the Author   233 •
Earn Continuing Education Credits/Units   234

Series Preface

Massage may be one of the oldest therapies still used today. At present more therapists than ever before are practicing an ever-expanding range of massage techniques. Many of these techniques are taught through massage schools and within degree courses. Our need now is to provide the best clinical and educational resources that will enable massage therapists to learn the required techniques for delivering massage therapy to clients. Human Kinetics has developed the Hands-On Guides for Therapists series with this in mind.

The Hands-On Guides for Therapists series provides specific tools of assessment and treatment that fall well within the realm of massage therapists but may also be useful for other bodyworkers, such as osteopaths and fitness instructors. Each book in the series is a step-by-step guide to delivering the techniques to clients. Each book features a full-colour interior packed with photos illustrating every technique. Tips provide handy advice to help you adjust your technique, and the Client Talk boxes contain examples of how the techniques can be used with clients who have particular problems. Throughout each book are questions that enable you to test your knowledge and skill, which will be particularly helpful if you are attempting to pass a qualification exam. We've even provided the answers too!

You might be using a book from the Hands-On Guides for Therapists series to obtain the required skills to help you pass a course or to brush up on skills you learned in the past. You might be a course tutor looking for ways to make massage therapy come alive with your students. This series provides easy-to-follow steps that will make the transition from theory to practice seem effortless. The Hands-On Guides for Therapists series is an essential resource for all those who are serious about massage therapy.

Over the years much has been written about hands-on, or manual, therapies. Techniques have been refined, reviewed and amended, promoting therapies as forms of art and not just simple protocols. Manual therapies today are acknowledged for making a difference in healthcare with even more therapists wanting to learn myofascial release (MFR).

For us, the manual therapist, the emergence of scientific discoveries that supports what we have been feeling under our hands provides a greater understanding and acceptance of what we do and how we do it.

MFR is a manual therapy used worldwide in a variety of treatment and rehabilitation approaches. Like massage, fascial and soft tissue work has grown and developed over the years. Once you grasp the fundamental theory and essential application of MFR, you soon realise that working with the entire fascial matrix (a three-dimensional web of tissue that supports, encompasses and protects every other structure in the body) is a process that is completely different from working just with the skin and muscles. This understanding differentiates not just this technique but the entire treatment approach from all other soft tissue approaches.

This is the second edition of *Myofascial Release*. It expands on the first edition by offering a blend of different MFR approaches that treat the entire body. The first edition discussed a comprehensive approach to sustained MFR. This second edition offers refinement expanding on essential MFR techniques, adding valuable and effective myofascial and soft tissue mobilisation techniques as well as treatments for scar tissue and adhesions. This new edition also comes with HK*Propel* access to online videos, which showcase visual demonstrations to help the reader learn the techniques.

This book describes MFR as a dynamic approach suitable for all students embarking on a career in hands-on therapy as well as for experienced therapists looking to add skills to their treatments. It also provides a greater understanding of the MFR approach for therapists who are already using fascial skills in their therapy sessions. Whether you are a physiotherapist or sports massage therapist or practise a complementary therapy for the whole body, this book describes MFR and shows how to apply the fundamental principles in your practice.

Many in healthcare today still struggle with the concept that no anatomical structure works in isolation and that body memory (the storage of information in the body, which is not limited to the brain) is an integral part of the healing process. Traditional healthcare often compartmentalises the workings of anatomy, and communication of a new paradigm among healthcare leaders and scientists can be challenging.

Myofascial therapists take time to listen to their clients and may be the only therapists who use their hands to feel for tissue dysfunction playing a contributing role in their client's pain and discomfort. Many people have undiagnosed pain and discomfort because fascial restrictions do not show up on regular hospital tests. Using MFR, a therapist is taught to feel for tissue restrictions and use appropriate techniques to resolve them. MFR provides an awareness of the dynamic and fluid fascial matrix on which all other structures depend.

Many therapists are looking for a therapy that provides physical and emotional results for their clients and is less harsh on their own hands and bodies. MFR offers unlimited possibilities to enhance therapists' present skills and to help them grow and expand their practices.

MFR is not a difficult therapy to learn. Through a refinement of kinaesthetic touch, results can be gained for both client and therapist. MFR is easily applied and provides results with minimal effort. Many mature therapists are drawn to MFR because it allows them to maintain their practices with less effort, whereas younger therapists gain a therapy that will provide them with longevity in their careers. MFR also does not require tools, oils or lotions. Because it is performed dry, skin on skin, it is easy to apply and prepare for.

Part I of this book provides the fundamental information you need to get started with MFR.

Chapter 1 describes what fascia and MFR are and discusses the benefits of MFR and how it differs from massage. Chapter 2 discusses the client consultation process and the subjective and objective assessments, whilst chapter 3 introduces contraindication for MFR, discusses the importance of the efficient and effective use of body mechanics and emphasises developing intuition and a sense of touch whilst cultivating fascial diagnostic and assessment skills.

Part II provides an overview of the techniques before diving into the details of each technique in part III. The techniques in part II span a wide range of effective MFR approaches. Many therapists will be familiar with techniques that use a slightly firmer pressure that I call myofascial mobilisations. These are akin to soft tissue release and pin and stretch techniques. However, the skill with these techniques is far more than the application process. It is practising the skill of kinaesthetic touch and becoming aware of the anatomy and tissue layers as they change beneath your hands. This skill is best learned from the other techniques in this part of the book, namely the cross-hand, transverse plane, and longitudinal pull techniques. These latter techniques are what are commonly called indirect sustained MFR techniques, and I encourage you to take time to practise these to increase your sense of touch.

Part III provides an easy guide and quick reference on commencing an MFR session, what to feel for, what the techniques are and how to perform them. This main part of the book details the MFR hands-on techniques and where on the body to apply them. Each set of techniques are described in detail so that you not only know where to apply them. Photographs support each technique showing body positioning and hand placement. As you work through the book, you will see that techniques integrate with each other with the ultimate goal of gaining a toolbox of effective techniques, so that each treatment you provide is unique to each client. Part IV describes how to further master MFR through combined and advanced techniques and how to develop specific treatment approaches. This part of the book showcases how to integrate your skill. It also gives you self-care applications so that you can add these to your treatments where clients can gain further benefit from a home-care MFR programme. I have offered suggestions of techniques which work well together, so that you can practise them as a group learning how to blend and mix and match techniques appropriately. Each chapter in the book also offers common, quick questions, the answers for which are found at the end of the book.

MFR is more than a technique; it is an entire therapeutic approach. More often than not, you will find that the best teachers are your clients; with this understanding, you will be prepared to learn something new every day. Few books exist on the entire MFR approach; most offer only the hands-on application. I have endeavoured to show that MFR depends on many processes, and to describe how to initiate some, how to integrate others, and how to follow, feel and listen to the client's body, all of which will allow you to use the techniques effectively. Like learning to drive, learning MFR takes time. This book offers valuable insights into this subject but will not make you an MFR therapist. However, it will get you well on your journey to using MFR effectively.

I hope this book offers a new and exciting way of working that is far more conducive to 'being with' your client as opposed to 'doing to' your client. I also hope that you do not simply find a new technique but a whole new way of working that will provide unlimited possibilities, thought-provoking experiences and an enjoyable, rewarding career.

Acknowledgements

It is often said that you never stop learning. This has certainly been the case with MFR. I started my journey with MFR two decades ago and still love learning from my students, clients and colleagues. There is no doubt that my own passion for the work was due to my own training from John F. Barnes, PT, and many of his skilled assistants in his treatment centres and seminars. John is a fantastic educator and therapist as well as a world leader in MFR. John's approach to MFR promotes a (w)holistic approach that treats the person, not the condition or injury.

I have attended many other MFR and soft tissue seminars also taught by highly experienced skilled manual therapists; I have loved them all. However, I have always had a soft spot for the sustained approach pioneered by John because it provides amazing results, resolving physical and emotional distress and pain.

Over the years I have developed my own way of working and have adapted many techniques, cultivating a blend of MFR specific to Myofascial Release UK (MFR UK). I will always give credit to my teachers, but John has been the most influential.

It has been seven years since the first edition of this book. In 2019, I attended a week's intensive treatment that was long overdue. My two highly skilled and experienced MFR therapists helped me find a new direction with my work and gave me the spark to write this second edition. These two therapists have always played a huge part in my MFR journey right from year one. Tina Matsuoka and June Greenberg, you are amazing. Thank you for always being there.

To Carol Davis, PT: Your quiet, thoughtful and considered approach to life, not just MFR, draws me even more to the work. You've taught me to stop, wait and feel and to accept that I can't fix everything. Your knowledge and passion to share MFR and the science of fascia is truly inspiring.

To the late Nancy Stewart, PT: Nancy was with me on the day I submitted the final draft of the first edition. I was typing madly to meet a deadline, and she just sat and drank tea. She was in the United Kingdom to teach a class on MFR for pelvic floor dysfunction for a group of advanced MFR therapists. Nancy had always been a huge supporter of my work and travelled to the United Kingdom on a number of occasions to teach for us. Nancy had acquired a huge knowledge base around cancer and fascia due to her own fight with leukaemia and myeloma. Nancy would email or video call me every time she had found something new. She was always interested in what I had learned and how our teaching was going. She encouraged me to keep going and to persevere. Nancy, I miss our chats.

Lastly, I couldn't have written this book without the amazing support, patience and enthusiasm of my close friends who share my passion for this work. You are always there, allowing me to use you as photo and video models, filling the gaps around assisting, packing vans and carrying boxes. To my 'prawn leg-warmers', you know who you are. Thank you for everything.

Getting Started With Myofascial Release

The first part of this book introduces the anatomy and function of the connective tissue system, which we call fascia. It describes different styles and techniques within the myofascial release (MFR) approach, how they work, what makes MFR different to other hands-on therapies and how it can benefit clients. Part I also addresses the important client consultation process, including checking for contraindications and performing the visual assessment. You will learn how to conduct some simple and informative palpatory assessments as well as how to prepare yourself and your environment for performing MFR.

Introduction to Myofascial Release

What is the myofascial system? *Myo* means 'muscle', and *fascia* means 'band'. Fascia, an embryologic tissue often sometimes called connective tissue, is a web-like, three-dimensional matrix that intertwines, surrounds, protects and supports every other structure of the human body. It is a single, uninterrupted sheet of tissue that extends from the inner aspects of the skull down to the soles of the feet and from the exterior to the interior of the body, ultimately making up the shape and form of the body itself.

Fascia has been described as the largest system in the human body because it touches all other structures and is said to be involved in the experience of pain (Pischinger 2007; Tesarz et al. 2011). On discussing the quantity of sensory nerve endings in fascia, Schleip (2021) reports that the entire fascial net has 50 million more nerve endings than the skin and over 120 million more sensory nerve endings than the eye. These figures demonstrate the reason as to why the fascial system has been promoted as a mechanosensitive signalling system with an integrated function akin to that of the nervous system (Langevin 2006). The fascial system is a totally integrated system and is the immediate environment of every cell in the body. This tensional network adapts its fibre arrangement and density according to the local and tensional demands placed on it (Schleip et al. 2012). The implications of this quality alone provide credibility for myofascial release (MFR) as well as scientific evidence of its significant role in health.

Only recently has the role of the fascial matrix been recognised. For many years the dissection process involved the complete discarding of the superficial fascia and failed to accept that the white fibrous tissue around muscles or the dynamic fluid web structures had any meaning, responsibility or role in health. Because fascial research is done on cadavers, the full potential of fascia is still unclear. However, recent filming of living fascia by Jean-Claude Guimberteau, a

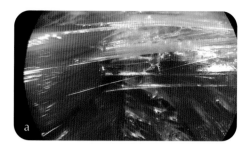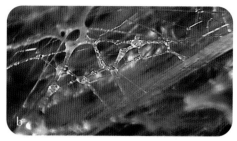

Figure 1.1   Fascia in vivo: *(a)* perimysium or muscle fascia, *(b)* fibrils in their subcutaneous sliding system. These images show fascia as a fluid-filled network extending throughout the entire body.

With kind permission of Dr. J.C. Guimberteau and Endovivo Productions. From *Endoscopic Anatomy of the Fascia,* by J. C. Guimberteau, MD, Handspring Publishing, 2014.

French hand surgeon, shows fascia as a dynamic, ever-changing, and adapting fluid-filled network present in and around every structure of the human body (see figure 1.1). Fascial restrictions do not show up on any traditional healthcare tests, yet MFR remains, and is increasingly, a much-sought-after therapy by both therapist and client.

The enormous amount of scientific research available on fascia now warrants an international congress held every two to three years that is attended by researchers, scientists, and therapists from all over the world. Research papers and general interest in fascia have dramatically increased during recent years and have promoted the benefits of fascial bodywork. Although a huge amount of fascial research, theory and scientific evidence is available, I will discuss only those aspects of fascia that I feel will help you understand the functions of fascia, its role in health and how myofascial approaches assist in restoring balance and function. Fascia has been aptly named the 'Cinderella of orthopaedic tissue' and has now become embraced, although initially very slowly, in the world of research and science; it is no longer viewed as a mere packing organ.

Elements of Fascia

Traditionally, when we discuss fascia, we are discussing the connective tissues of the muscular system. However, a more encompassing definition was developed at the 2012 International Fascial Congress in Vancouver, Canada. The term *fascia* now describes not only the muscular fascia of the endomysium, perimysium and epimysium, but all of the soft tissue components of the connective tissue system that permeate the human body forming part of the body-wide tensional force transmission system. Therefore, fascia now also includes the aponeurosis, ligaments, tendons, joint capsules, and certain layers of bone, organs and nerves, as well as the dura mater surrounding the central nervous system, the epineurium (i.e., a fascial layer around peripheral nerves) and bronchial connective tissues and the mesentery of the abdomen (Huijing and Langevin 2009).

The terminological clarification, or nomenclature, was a huge topic of debate at the 2015 Fascia Research Congress in Washington, D.C., where Carla Stecco, MD, announced that a general nomenclature committee had been set up to define the fascia in line with Federative International Programme of Anatomical Terminologies (FIPAT), which has led to the anatomical definition of fascia as

> a sheath, a sheet or any number of other dissectible aggregations of connective tissue that forms beneath the skin to attach, enclose, separate muscles and other internal organs. (Stecco and Schleip 2016)

However, this definition was purely from the anatomical point of view, and it received criticism from practitioners and clinicians. A further subcommittee has now established a clinical definition for the fascial system as follows.

> The fascial system consists of the three-dimensional continuum of soft, collagen containing, loose and dense fibrous connective tissues that permeate the body. It incorporates elements such as adipose tissue, adventitia and neurovascular sheaths, aponeuroses, deep and superficial fasciae, epineurium, joint capsules, ligaments, membranes, meninges, myofascial expansions, periostea, retinacula, septa, tendons, visceral fasciae, and all the intramuscular and intermuscular connective tissues including endo-/peri-/epimysium. The fascial system surrounds, interweaves between, and interpenetrates all organs, muscles, bones and nerve fibers, endowing the body with a functional structure, and providing an environment that enables all body systems to operate in an integrated manner. (Stecco et al. 2018)

The fascial web spreads three-dimensionally throughout the body as it enfolds and embraces all other soft tissue and organs. No tissue exists in isolation; all act on, and are bound and interwoven with, other structures. Through its continuity, the fascial web forms supportive structures to maintain hydrostatic pressure, promoting the visceral function of and protecting the vital organs.

Fascia enfolds the muscular system and osseous structures connecting muscles, tendons, joints and bones. In fact, it could be argued that there is no such thing as 'a' muscle because fascia binds and connects every muscle—the fibril, fascicle and fibre—to the next, and to all other structures, acting as a continuous tensile network.

Like muscles, fascia also is sensitive to mechanical loads. The sensory mechanoreceptors of fascia, receptors that respond to mechanical load or distortion, are stimulated in different ways offering further scope to the refinement of MFR treatment and rehabilitation. The Golgi tendon organs respond to active stretch and pressure, the Pacini and Ruffini corpuscles respond to rapid pressure changes and vibrational movements whilst the Ruffini also responds to sustained pressure and tangential stretch. Lastly, the interstitial free nerve endings respond to both rapid and sustained pressure changes (Schleip et al. 2012).

These interstitial free nerve endings are polymodal. That is, they transmit more than one type of afferent message from the fascia to the central nervous system. These fibres convey nociceptive, thermoreceptive and interoceptive information in unmyelinated nerves transmitting information on potential or actual tissue injury, temperature changes and the awareness of the sense of self respectively (Schleip 2017).

Research on fascia suggests that muscles hardly ever transmit the full force of their strength through their tendons onto bone attachments. Rather, force is distributed onto both tendon and the fascial network, distributing this force to associated fascial sheaths, synergistic and antagonistic muscles, nearby joints and other structures (Findlay, Chaudhry and Dhar, 2015). This understanding renders the concept of lever actions and specific muscles being responsible for certain actions somewhat incomplete.

Fascia is dynamic because it constantly changes. It continually morphs in response to the demands of both the internal and external tension imposed on it. The human framework depends on this single tensional network of connective tissue. We would not be able to exist without this ever-adapting, gel-filled network maintaining our integrity with every breath we take.

Collagen and Elastin

Collagen is the most abundant protein in the body. Both collagen and elastin, another type of protein, are the main fibres within fascia, and together they exist within a viscous, gel-like fluid called ground substance. The specific composition of fascia is determined by its role in the body; it forms in a variety of ways depending on its function. Collagen provides strength and stability when mechanical stress is applied, to guard against overextension. Elastin provides an elastic quality that allows the connective tissue to stretch to the limit of the collagen fibres' length whilst absorbing tensile force.

Fascia is a colloid, which is a continually changing substance defined by stability, attraction forces and repulsion forces of molecules in close proximity to each other. A colloid comprises particles of solid material suspended in fluid (e.g., wallpaper paste) (Chaitow, 2018). Colloids are not rigid; they conform to the shape of their containers and respond to pressure even though they are not compressible. The amount of resistance colloids offers increases proportionally to the velocity of force applied to them. The more rapidly force is applied, the more rigid the tissue becomes. This is why a gentle, light, sustained touch is essential to avoid resistance and viscous drag when releasing fascial restrictions.

Ground Substance

Surrounding the collagen and elastin fibres is a viscous, gel-like ground substance (a polysaccharide gel complex) composed of hyaluronic acid (hyaluronan, or HA) and proteoglycans that lubricate the fibres and allow them to glide over each other (Barnes 1990, p. 3; Chaitow and DeLany 2008, p. 1). The ground substance is the immediate environment for all the cells in the body. The proteoglycans form this gel-like medium, and the presence of the HA, secreted by a specialised fascial cell called a fasciacyte, makes it hydrophilic (water loving), drawing water into the tissue (Stecco et al. 2018). This provides a cushioning effect as well as main-taining space and tissue glide between the collagen fibres. The gel absorbs shock and disperses it throughout the body. A contributing factor of fascial dysfunction is the increase of viscosity of the ground substance, which thus limits fascial glide.

Fascia's ground substance provides the medium in which other elements are exchanged (gases, nutrients, hormones, cellular waste, antibodies and white blood cells). The condition of the ground substance can affect the rate of diffusion and therefore the health of the cells it surrounds (Chaitow and DeLany 2008, p. 1; Juhan 2003, p. 59).

Elastic Properties and Force Transmission

Fascia, like other soft tissue and biological structures, has an innate, variable degree of elasticity that allows it to withstand deformation when forces and pressures are applied to it. It can then recover and return to its starting shape and size. Because fascia contracts and relaxes, it responds to load, compression and force. At the beginning of loading, fascia has an elastic response in which a degree of slack is taken up.

Over time, if loading persists in a slow and sustained manner, creep develops, which is a slow, delayed yet continuous deformation. Subsequently, an actual volume change occurs as water is forced from the tissue (i.e., the ground substance becomes less gel-like).

When the applied force, or loading, ceases, fascia should return to its original non-deformed state. The restoration of shape occurs through elastic recoil via hysteresis, the process of energy use and loss in which tissues are loaded and unloaded. The time needed for tissue to return to normal via elastic recoil depends on the uptake of water by the tissue and whether its elastic potential has been exceeded. When loaded for any length of time, tissues lengthen and distort until they reach a point of balance. If loading is sustained, over time chronic deformation will result.

Fascia responds to pressure both internally and externally and transmits that force throughout its matrix. This tensional force transmission system can be viewed as a tensegrity model. *Tensegrity*, a combination of the words *tension* and *integrity*, is a term coined by Buckminster Fuller, an American architect, designer and inventor. Tensegrity, or tensional integrity, refers to a form of integrity that is based on a balance between tension and compression. Biological structures such as muscle, soft tissue and bone are made strong by a combination of tensioned and compressed parts. The musculoskeletal system is a synergy of muscle, soft tissue and bone; the muscle and soft tissue provide continuous pull whilst the bones provide discontinuous push.

Muscle and Fascia Connections

Connective tissue (fascia) provides support for more highly organised structures and attaches extensively to muscle. Individual muscle fibres are enveloped by endomysium, which is connected to the stronger perimysium, which surrounds the fasciculi. The perimysium fibres attach to the even stronger epimysium, which surrounds the muscle as a whole and attaches to the fascial tissues nearby.

Because connective tissue contains mesenchymal cells of an embryonic type, it is generalised in a way that makes it capable of giving rise, under certain circumstances, to more specialised elements. It forms the periosteum around the bone, the pericardium around the heart, the pleura around the lungs, the fascial sheath around every digestive organ and the synovial sheaths around every tendon, and it is thickened to form the various protective retinacula throughout the body.

Muscle and fascia are anatomically inseparable; fascia moves in response to muscle activity. Many of the neural structures in fascia are sensory in nature. Fascia is critically involved in proprioception, which is essential for postural integrity (Langevin 2006). Research shows that numerous myelinated neural structures relating to both proprioception and pain reception exist in fascia. After joint and muscle spindle input is taken into account, the majority of the remaining proprioception occurs in the fascial sheaths.

Fascia supplies restraining mechanisms by the differentiation of retention bands, fibrous pulleys and check ligaments and also assists in the harmonious production and control of movement. Specialised fascia is interwoven with tendinous and ligamentous structures and enables adjacent tissues to move upon each other whilst providing stability. When in a healthy, well-lubricated state, fascia ensures that adjacent structures glide against each other allowing free movement. It enhances the body's postural balance allowing for free and efficient movement. The ensheathing layers of deep fascia, as well as the intermuscular septum and the interosseous membranes, provide vast areas used for muscular attachment.

Fascial Force Transmission

We are taught that muscles act over joints and rarely transmit their entire force through muscle alone. Rather, force is transmitted through fascial sheathing (epimysium and perimysium) surrounding muscles and joints. Muscles are therefore part of the continuous tensile fascial network. This transfer of force, called force transmission, offers new insight into body-wide dysfunction and to total-body rehabilitation regardless of the site of pain and injury.

The fascial continuity creates a direct relationship between muscular synergists and antagonists where the permeating and surrounding fascia contribute to approximately 30 percent of force transmission (Huijing, Maas and Baan 2003). Fascia is not only involved in moving joints, but assists in muscular coordination, control and the transmission of force to antagonists and associated biokinetic chains in order to maintain balance in the gravitational field (Huijing 2007). Research has shown that fascia creates a radial stress to the muscle, shortening the muscle and bringing the tendons closer together (Findlay, Chaudhry and Dhar, 2015).

This new view of force transmission is a paradigm shift from the linear view of biomechanics to incorporating biotensegrity promoting a more holistic approach. This radial stress can also become dysfunctional, affecting muscle action. MFR techniques can be applied to muscle in both longitudinal and transverse manners to restore muscle function.

Fascia also has the potential for elastic recoil and energy storage. Fascia is dominantly shaped by tensional strain opposed to compression and is intricately connected to muscle. Fascia can absorb force along its entire network and use that force to great potential along with muscular coordination.

Fascia and Cellular Elements

Fascia provides a course for interstitial fluid and in so doing provides lubrication between structures to allow for movement and the delivery of nutrition. The meshes of loose connective tissue contain the tissue fluid that provides an essential medium through which cellular elements of other tissues are brought into functional relation with blood and lymph. This occurs partly by diffusion and partly by hydrokinetic transportation encouraged by alterations in pressure gradients (e.g., between the thorax and the abdominal cavity during inhalation and exhalation). Connective tissue has a nutritive function and houses nearly a quarter of all body fluids.

The histiocytes of connective tissue play an important defensive role against bacterial invasion by their phagocytic activity. Fluid and infectious processes often travel along the fascial planes. They also act as scavengers by removing cell debris and foreign material. Connective tissue also is an important neutraliser, or detoxicant, of both endogenous toxins (those produced under physiological conditions) and exogenous toxins. The anatomical barrier presented by fascia has important defensive functions in case of infections and toxaemia.

The more we learn about fascia, the more we understand how important it is to the function of every cell of the body. In addition to providing support, protection and the separation of structural elements, as discussed, fascia plays a vital role in the following functions:

- Cellular respiration
- Elimination
- Metabolism
- Fluid and lymph flow
- Repair by deposition of repair tissue
- Conservation of body heat
- Fat storage
- Cellular health and the immune system

Superficial and Deep Fascia

The new definition of fascia addresses the superficial (see figure 1.2a) and deep (see figure 1.2b) fascial layers, which can be distinguished by trained hands. These two layers and their associated structures are enveloped within the global fascial matrix and are therefore in complete communication with each other. Imagine that your body is knitted three-dimensionally, and within that knitted framework are your bones, muscles, nerves, vessels, organs, brain and all the other structures of your body. Without fascia, your body would not have form, function or support.

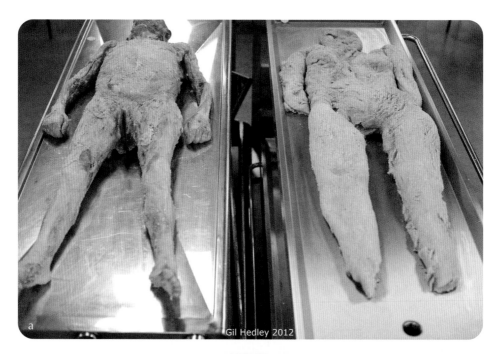

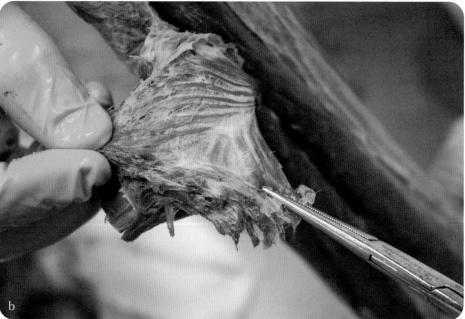

Figure 1.2   *(a)* The entire superficial fascia of an adult woman dissected in order to demonstrate its size and role in body shape and contour. *(b)* Deep fascia visible between layers of the gastrocnemius muscle of the lower leg.

(a) With kind permission of Gil Hedley, PhD, and Integral Anatomy Productions, LLC. *(b)* With kind permission of Julian Baker and Functional Fascia Ltd.

Superficial fascia

- forms a thin layer of tissue beneath the skin, attaching the dermis skin to the underlying tissues;
- provides shock absorption;
- is loosely knit;
- consists of fibroelastic, areolar tissue;
- provides space for the accumulation of fluid and metabolites;
- stores fat;
- provides insulation;
- contains capillary networks and lymphatic channels;
- regulates fluid;
- contains inflammatory exudates; and
- causes many tissue texture abnormalities.

Deep fascia

- is tough, tight and compact;
- contributes to the contour and function of the body;
- comprises the specialised elements of the peritoneum, pericardium and pleura;
- forms many interconnected pockets;
- has tough, inelastic clefts and septa;
- compartmentalises the entire muscular system;
- surrounds and separates visceral organs;
- thickens in response to stress;
- functions posturally to stabilise; and
- encases the nervous system and the brain.

The tough, resistant and confining nature of deep fascia can create problems such as the compartment syndromes. Trauma with haemorrhage in the anterior compartment of the lower leg can cause swelling that is detrimental to the sensitive neural structures within the compartments. Frequently, fasciectomy is necessary to relieve the compression on the neural elements.

The visceral fascia surrounds and supports the organs by wrapping them in layers of connective tissue. Postural adaptations, injury and trauma, including surgery of any kind, have a detrimental effect on these fine layers of fascia. Adhesions in the visceral fascia can affect organ function, including digestion and elimination, as well as create pain and discomfort. A skilled MFR therapist can detect these adhesions and gently separate them, restoring function and eliminating pain.

Conditions That Affect Fascia

Fascia shortens, solidifies and thickens, a process called densification, in response to trauma, anything physically or emotionally injurious to the body, inflammation and poor posture, causing the body to lose its physiological adaptive capacity. In general we call this a 'binding down' of fascia. Deformation and distortion of any part of this network imposes negative stresses on distant aspects and on the structures it divides, envelopes, enmeshes and supports, and with which it connects. This alone can alter organ and tissue significantly. The densification and binding down of the tissues is also compounded by the increased viscosity of the ground substance negatively impacting the global network.

Over time, fascial restrictions insidiously spread like a pull in a sweater or stocking. Flexibility and spontaneity of movement are lost, setting up the body for more trauma, pain and movement limitation. Although fascia is predominantly aligned top to toe, abnormal forces can cause it to twist and turn, increasing the tensile force and pulling the body out of its three-dimensional alignment with the vertical gravitation axis. This results in biomechanical inefficiency and highly energy-consuming movement and posture. Deformation of tissues and the tensile force of the entire fascial unit can create pressure of up to 2,000 pounds per square inch on pain-sensitive structures (Katake 1961).

As the fascial network binds down, it creates restriction not only in the area of injury but also throughout its entire structure, affecting both adjacent and distant pain-sensitive structures. This results in unique adaptations that eventually become like a scrapbook of traumatic events, somewhat like a holographic imprint. The three primary conditions that cause fascia to bind down are injury, inflammation and poor posture.

Injury or Trauma

The body can become injured from an event such as a fall, blow, cut or burn as well as when the body systems become dysfunctional for one reason or another. Injury also includes surgery scarring and adhesions of any kind, the effects of medication and overuse and underuse of the tissues as in a sporting injury. Trauma refers to any kind of injury or hurt whether physical, emotional or spiritual. Many people experience traumatic events as children that cause them to react and act in certain ways. These childlike, and sometimes childish, reactions and actions are carried into adulthood where they are further complicated by the general stresses of daily life.

Inflammatory Processes

The fascial system can be compromised by an inflammatory response to injury, a medical condition or the side effects from medication. The inflammatory response creates an imbalance in cellular fluids and possible cell death from lack of oxygen, resulting in scar formation and fascial adhesions.

Habitually Poor Posture

Postural adaptations refer to how we place ourselves in positions to perform tasks or to cope with strain or stress that can be either physical or emotional. When performed long enough, these adaptations become unconscious and we adopt them automatically, not realising that we may be injuring our bodies.

When fascia is consistently overloaded from supporting a position in space (standing, seated or lying), it has to bind down and densify to support the pressure imposed on it. As it deforms, an abnormal pull is created (i.e., it binds down), which in turn creates further postural imbalance, worsening the condition. Because this imbalance occurs over a long time, the person usually doesn't realise it until it is too late.

Muscles are injured at a point somewhere between their origin and insertion. Fascia, however, has no end point; it is completely continuous. For this reason, the site of the original injury, physical and emotional, can be the cause of further injuries that quietly creep through the entire fascial system and become compensatory patterns that promote further injuries or conditions that seem to have no connection to the original trauma.

Osseous structures are passive elements and are influenced by the soft tissue supporting them. Restricted fascial strain patterns can crowd or pull the osseous structures out of proper alignment, resulting in the compression of joints and producing pain or dysfunction, or both.

As fascia binds down, myofascial theory promotes that it is not only the physical structures that become restricted; the thoughts, memory and reactions that were felt at the time of injury also become restricted. We call this body memory. When body memory becomes stuck, it replays the same message over and over again, long after the actual event is over. This frozen moment in time produces the effect described in Hans Selye's work (1955) on the general adaptation syndrome of alarm and reaction, a state of resistance followed by a state of exhaustion. Neural and vascular structures can also become trapped in these restrictions, causing neurological or ischemic conditions. Moreover, shortening of the myofascial fascicle can limit its functional length, reducing its strength, contractile potential and deceleration capacity.

Fascia is your anti-gravity system, responding to stress by absorbing and distributing it along its entire network to maintain balance and reduce both physical and emotional trauma to a minimum. Restrictions of any nature promote further injury. A combination of physical and emotional trauma (in fact, they should never be separated) with added time, pressure and stress, describes the vast majority of conditions we see in clients today.

The fascial network constantly tries to compensate, communicating the tension throughout its entire network and working as a unit to attempt to offer strain- and pain-free function using the least amount of energy. The more dysfunction there is, the less dynamic fascia becomes, and instead of maintaining structural integrity, fascia becomes so restricted that it causes structural deformation instead. Restrictions present at the time of trauma prevent any other forces or pressures from being dispersed properly. As a result, areas of the body are subject to an intolerable impact, and injury occurs. Compensations through muscular spasm and fascial restrictions ultimately produce symptoms.

Myofascial Release Concepts

MFR has origins in soft tissue or myofascial mobilisation, osteopathy, physical therapy, craniosacral therapy and energy work, among others, and all have become subtly blended to form what has been known as myofascial release for a number of decades.

MFR is not massage in that it uses no lubrication (oil, cream or lotion) to avoid slipping on the skin. Rather, the therapist employs 'listening hands' to feel for tissue tension followed by skilled touch that, without forcing the tissue, addresses tight and tender areas in the body. MFR applications are always slow and diligent and are kept within patient tolerance levels. The skills to the MFR application are patience, intuition and a heightened kinaesthetic touch.

MFR is not a new therapy; evidence of its beginnings can be found in the work of osteopath Andrew Taylor Still around the turn of the 19th century. However, the term *myofascial* was not commonly used until the 1960s and '70s when Janet Travell and David Simons revolutionised the understanding of referred pain with their theory of myofascial trigger points, which highlighted the potential cause of muscle pain and dysfunction. However, MFR is more than a treatment for trigger points; it is a therapy that actively treats the tissue tension and dysfunction contributing to generalised myofascial pain, which may include trigger point formation.

According to some reports, the term 'myofascial release' was first used at a soft tissue course taught at Michigan State University in 1981; however, more commonly, the term has been pioneered in the United States by John F. Barnes, a physical therapist who has been actively teaching his own style of the sustained, often called the indirect, approach to MFR since the 1980s. Barnes has played a major role as an MFR educator over the last few decades, and scientific research now supports his approach as a valuable treatment for fascial dysfunction.

Resent Research Findings

Dr Gerald Pollack's research regarding the water content of fascia highlights the huge role of fluid dynamics in fascial bodywork. This research proposes that water has another state beside gaseous, frozen and liquid: that of a gel. He also describes water as having two main states, bound water and free water. Water, in the presence of a hydrophilic (water-loving) tissue, organises itself in a colloidal matrix of particles that forms a liquid crystal. Pollack describes this liquid crystal as bound water. Bound water has a high degree of viscoelasticity, giving it a trampoline-like bounce and give. Free water is more chaotic in its organisation and is charged differently to bound water (Pollack 2013, p. 281).

The protein collagen is a hydrophilic tissue. Water, which makes up approximately two thirds of fascial composition, in proximity to collagen forms bound water, which promotes the bounce and give that enhances nutrient, gaseous, waste product and information exchange. In restricted fascia, however, in which the collagen and elastin fibres are drawn closer together, less bound water is present. Elastin is a hydrophobic (water-hating) tissue that pushes the bound water (created by the hydrophilic collagen fibres) away from it, leaving its free water to initiate and maintain inflammatory processes.

Pollack goes on to describes how photonic energy (electromagnetic radiation) charges bound water, increasing its viscoelasticity and promoting a healthier tissue tone. Photonic energy is present everywhere, including in infrared energy (heat), which is present in and transmitted through the therapist's hands into the client's body during MFR. This confirms Barnes' theory that the fascial gel, or ground substance, can be influenced by water exchange through the slow and sustained pressure of trained hands.

Bhowmick et al. (2009), Meltzer et al. (2010) and Standley and Metzer (2008) have also produced interesting research. Bhowmick et al. address the role of fascia on the immune system, in particular the T3 cells. During the sympathetic fight-or-flight response a substance called transforming growth factor beta (TGF-beta) is released into the fascial network and has been found to be responsible for fascial tonicity. TGF-beta is a potent stimulator of myofibroblast contraction, wound contracture and scar tissue and fibrosis creation, all of which negatively affect the immune system, making fascial tissue feel more restricted and less bouncy. MFR, with its slow, sustained pressure, influences the autonomic nervous system, creating a mental and manual shift from the sympathetic fight-or-flight response to the parasympathetic rest and digest tone, counteracting TGF-beta and improving immune system response. Meltzer and colleagues' research focuses on interleukin, a cytokine crystalline communicatory protein that promotes healing. They showed reduced levels of interleukin with fascial holds of less than three minutes. Interleukin 8, which regulates inflammatory responses, was not stimulated until fascial holds reached three minutes, and it more than doubled at five-minute holds. Interleukin 3, which regulates blood cell production, increased after four-minute fascial holds (Meltzer et al. 2010).

> continued

> continued

Research from Fede et al. (2016) discusses hormone receptor expression in human fascia with a potential link to an increased level of myofascial pain and tissue fibrosis in post-menopausal women as a result of a decline in oestrogen. Another insight into the aetiology of myofascial pain is discussed by Stecco et al. (2011), who hypothesise that the increased levels of HA secreted by the fasciacytes increases viscosity and contributes to the lack of gliding between the deep fascia and muscle and also between the loose connective tissues. Menon et al. (2020) discuss not only the potential role of HA in myofascial pain due to its increased viscosity but also the use of imaging enhancement of an MRI scanner capable of targeting the presence of a higher concentration of HA, which may further confirm the function of fascia's role in the pain experience.

Other pioneers include Dr Ida P. Rolf, a biochemist who established the soft tissue manipulation and movement programme called Rolfing. Rolfing is far more popular in North America than in Europe, with many therapists offering Rolf's 10-step approach to health. Thomas Myers, a student of Rolf, continues with much of her work in his Anatomy Trains method of structural integration. Art Riggs, Robert Schleip, James Waslaski, Erik Dalton, Noah Karrasch, James Earls and many other well-known manual therapy educators follow Rolf's approach to MFR. Routinely, this style of MFR is called the direct approach because Rolf said it 'takes the tissue to where it ain't.' The direct approach has many names including soft tissue release (STR), soft tissue or myofascial mobilisation, active release therapy (ART), pin and stretch, and lever techniques. Additionally, in some countries, direct MFR is also known as deep tissue massage or deep tissue release therapy.

The direct approach, that I will call myofascial mobilisation, uses fingers, knuckles, elbows and thumbs applied to the tissue at an oblique angle, moving slowly along muscle and muscle chains or lines from either muscle insertion to origin or vice versa. The therapist can also apply pressure in multiple directions across the muscle and muscle chains because the fascial system has been shown to be involved in muscular contraction, assisting in expansion of the circumference of the muscle.

This application is slightly firmer than the sustained approach to MFR but is always applied within client tolerance. Often, the client actively moves the limb or body part being treated, or the therapist can move the limb or body part in a passive movement.

It's of value here to note that the term 'myofascial release' is not owned by anyone just as the term massage is not owned by anyone either. Many educators label their MFR approach using their own name as Ida P. Rolf did with Rolfing which is trademarked. Others simply say that they teach their own approach to MFR as John F. Barnes has done. This means that you will find educators teaching MFR, but they have named it to be more specific to themselves or what they believe they are doing to the tissue.

There is also some criticism of the word release when discussing MFR. What are we actually releasing, and can that actually be done? To release something suggests that it is let go of such as releasing a bird from a cage. The late Leon Chaitow, DO, discussed this issue in his article 'What's in a name: Myofascial Release or Myofascial Induction?' (Chaitow, 2017). As fascia has a supporting and protecting role, the word release isn't really correct. Furthermore, releasing pain isn't accurate either as pain is not stored in the body. Releasing scar tissue and restrictions can't really be physically done either unless by a scalpel. While I agree that the word *release* isn't the right word when trying to describe the physiological effects of MFR, I think we need to look at it from a far more subjective point of view. I do think that it is very logical and appropriate to say that we are releasing the client's perception of their pain and tension. Far too often these days we feel forced to look at evidence-based approaches to gain credibility. However, the narrative approach, which is listening to the client, supporting them and releasing what they feel is holding them hostage I think is far more important. If MFR can be used to help clients regain a healthy pain-free life, then changing its name is irrelevant.

New knowledge of the fascia and its role supports the use of MFR for the treatment of the body-wide fascial network, as opposed to only the myofascia (the fascia in and around muscles), which is addressed more commonly with the direct approach. The indirect sustained approach uses the position of ease of the tissues, not forcing any tissue past that position of ease. The sustained indirect approach also embraces the concept of 'find the pain and look elsewhere for the cause', a quote often used by John F. Barnes in his MFR seminars. This approach uses slow, lighter pressure from flat hands or the side of the arm, gently sinking into and following the tissue, waiting patiently at the tissue end range for it to change and yield in response to the subtle gentle pressure. The techniques are applied for approximately three to five minutes to allow for tissue and nervous system reorganisation.

Finally, the indirect sustained form of MFR has become an acceptable manual therapy playing a valuable role in the restoration of health and well-being for those suffering from conditions such as PTSD. While additional training should be completed to obtain specialist skills to work with PTSD and other emotional disorders, many therapists will eventually specialise in using MFR to assist clients with both physical and emotional issues.

However, despite the application of MFR having two quite separate camps in the application, it is far more useful to view and use MFR as a totally integrated manual therapy approach, blending all styles of MFR together to meet the physical and mental needs of the client. Having the knowledge, understanding and skill of MFR as an integrated approach offers a greater scope for treatment efficacy. From this viewpoint, MFR becomes not only a treatment but also a rehabilitation and self-care approach.

The therapist applies pressure with their hands onto, and into, the client's body, requesting client feedback to actively engage the client in the process. In this way MFR is a client-led therapy. The therapist addresses the tissue barrier of resistance by feeling for tightness, restrictions and adhesions in any plane that may be causing pain or dysfunction.

Generally, clients are treated in their underwear or shorts and a bra top with sheets or towels for drapes. In most cases the MFR therapist performs a visual, movement and palpatory assessment and obtains a client consultation form.

Once the evaluation has been completed, the therapist commences treatment in areas that feel tight, hot or tender. These areas will not always be where the client is experiencing pain. This is because MFR is based on the entire fascial matrix, which, when restricted, creates a tensile force, affecting pain-sensitive structures throughout its network.

Imagine standing at one end of a long banquet table covered in a tablecloth and taking hold of the corners of the tablecloth. Pulling equally on both corners, you pull the tablecloth towards you evenly. Now imagine that the tablecloth has a nail driven into the middle and slightly to the right side of the table. If you take hold of the corners of the tablecloth again and pull, you won't be able to pull evenly; in fact, the harder you pull, the tighter the cloth becomes. Now imagine that the corners of the tablecloth you are pulling are the areas of pain and where the nail is, is the restricted fascia. The more you work with the site of pain, stretching and releasing the tissue, the more give the restricted area has to bind the tissue towards it. However, if you follow those lines of restriction back to the origin (i.e., the nail) and remove it, you can restore the entire structure to an even and equal pull. This is how MFR works on a three-dimensional level. You take note of where the pain is, but you look, feel and trace the restricted tissue back to its origin, then work with creating balance and restoring function using appropriate MFR techniques.

The actual application of the hands-on technique is a slow, sustained pressure held at the barrier of tissue resistance until a sensation of melting is perceived by the therapist. Depending on the body area, the therapist might slowly and diligently lean into the tissue with the hand, elbow or loose fist, gliding through the tissue. Concurrently, active or passive movement of the tissue or limb can also be done to encourage tissue change. Alternatively, a sustained pressure is held at the barrier of tissue resistance usually for three to five minutes or more without slipping over the skin. The viscoelastic nature of fascia causes it to resist sudden forces. The Arndt-Schultz law, which states that weak stimuli increase physiological activity and very strong stimuli inhibit or abolish activity, shows that less is more. Less pressure applied to tissue results in a greater response; firmer and quicker pressure results in tissue resistance. This emphasises the need for slow, sustained pressure, not forgetting the response of the various mechanoreceptors. If you push a boat away from a dock quickly, the boat digs into the water and doesn't go very far. However, if you apply a gentle force, meeting the resistance of the water, the boat will drift farther away. MFR works the same way.

MFR therapists learn to become highly sensitive to the ebb and flow of the tissues under their hands by applying gently sustained pressure. Imagine that tissue is like a sponge. An MFR therapist slowly squeezes out the free water from the tissue, encouraging fresh, clean water to return. At the same time, the hydrophilic nature of the collagen encourages the water molecules to organise themselves in the liquid crystalline matrix form, which Pollack calls bound water. The colloidal liquid crystalline matrix of bound water provides it with a high degree of viscoelasticity, promoting bounce and give within the system.

The four mechanoreceptors of the fascial matrix mentioned earlier, Golgi, Pacini, Ruffini and the interstitial free nerve endings (Schleip et al. 2012) respond to stimuli. MFR, through its cultivation of touch and kinaesthetic awareness, stimulates these mechanoreceptors by applying pressure-sensitive techniques followed by sustained pressure to influence fascial tonicity change.

It is thought that the time needed for tissues to begin to rearrange themselves is approximately 90 to 120 seconds; the viscous ground substance determines the ease at which this occurs. Because collagen begins to change only after 90 to 120 seconds, MFR techniques must be performed for more than five minutes to influence the entire fascial network (Barnes 1990). MFR is also thought to influence the collagen and elastin fibres to rearrange themselves into a more conducive resting length by the application of biomechanical energy or pressure from the therapist's hands (piezoelectricity). This makes use of the semiconductive nature of proteins.

As the collagen and elastin fibres reorganise themselves, cross-linkages in these fibres are broken down, fascial planes are realigned, local circulation (waste and nutrient exchange) improves and the soft tissue proprioceptive sensory mechanisms are reset. As the sensory mechanisms are reset, there is a reprogramming of the central nervous system, enabling a normal functional range of motion without eliciting the old pain pattern.

Taking into consideration the viscoelastic nature of fascia, its mechanoreceptive properties and the Arndt-Schultz law, it becomes clear that the application of quick, firm force will result in the entire matrix effectively pushing the therapist's hands back out. Instead, the therapist must place the hands on the body and, with a gentle pressure, lean into the tissue to reach the barrier of restriction. The feeling of the various fascial layers is quite distinguishable to trained hands, which is discussed later. The therapist waits, feeling for the moment the hands sink into the tissue, and takes up the slack as it is offered. The time element is important. The slower the pressure is applied, the greater the change within the viscoelastic ground substance. The slow, sustained pressure also allows the therapist to connect with the entire fascial matrix, increasing the kinaesthetic awareness of restrictions that may be distant to where the hands are; these restrictions draw the hands towards them.

Apart from the physiological response to pressure applied for about 90 to 120 seconds is the fact that the system recognises the pressure as a positive influence. Fascia responds to touch by softening and yielding, allowing the therapist to follow that softening through barrier after barrier of restriction in any direction in a three-dimensional manner. This sensitivity of the fascial restrictions in all planes and the yielding of the tissue to the sustained pressure applied without force and without slipping on the skin creates an environment in which the time element and kinaesthetic awareness of each technique is paramount.

MFR therapists feel for tissue resistance in all techniques; this is called the end-feel, or tissue barrier. The term *end-feel* is used to refer to where the tissue moves and where is it stuck. Where it feels stuck (i.e., has an abnormal end-feel) is where a technique is applied; the client is then re-assessed and treated accordingly. In MFR the end-feel is where the tissue (fascia) feels stuck and is resistive to subtle pressure or traction. If the therapist continues to pull or push (i.e., force) past this tissue resistance, or end-feel, the tissue simply shuts down and the efforts to treat it become useless.

The MFR therapist may complete two or three fascial techniques and then have the client stand up again so the therapist can see and feel what has changed and where to treat next. Another important form of feedback during the treatment session, to help the therapist determine technique progression, is vasodilation, or red flare. This occurs where there is an increase in circulation as the tissue reorganises along the lines of pull. The client may also report a sense of tissue movement or softening in sites distant to where the therapist's hands are. This is thought to result from the change to the tissue tension and from the receptive fields of the somatosensory system.

As mentioned earlier, less is more with MFR. It is not about how much pressure you use; it's about how much resistance you feel. Because everyone's fascial makeup is unique, the work has to be applied as a unique, individualised treatment. People are injured three-dimensionally in space and have three-dimensional bodies. Therefore, you must treat them with the pressure their own unique fascial matrix requires, in a three-dimensional manner.

One last key aspect of the MFR approach is encouraging clients to increase their awareness of their own body. This state of self-awareness encourages interoception. Interoception is the awareness of the physiological condition of the body and includes the sense of itch, tickle, sensual touch, visceral sensations, hunger and thirst (Craig 2003). Fascia's free nerve endings play a major role in conveying interoceptive awareness to the brain, where the lack of interoceptive awareness is linked to stress, anxiety and depression (Schleip 2012). Thus, in actively encouraging the client to feel the sensations in their body from MFR, they increase their interoceptive awareness. Additionally, research presented at the 2012 International Fascia Research Congress showed that sensory stimulation is enhanced by active cortical stimulation (Moseley, Zalucki and Wiech 2008). In other words, actively engaging the client in the treatment process using therapeutic dialoguing increases therapy results.

CLIENT TALK

Many therapists ask what the best MFR techniques are for a particular symptom or injury. If a client presents with recurring pain or a symptom, we should view the body as a whole, moving out of symptomatic treatment to that of creating total-body balance and function. We have to accept the fact that each part of the body is responsible for supporting and creating integrity for all its counterparts; no one part lives in isolation (tensegrity). As a consequence, no specific techniques exist for specific aches, pains or injuries. A client who has a repetitive shoulder injury will never find resolution if his ribcage, pelvis and ankles are not functioning or balanced properly because these structures support the shoulder. The same process applies to conditions such as fibromyalgia and chronic fatigue syndrome. Although the symptoms may be similar from client to client, the reasons the symptoms are elicited may be completely different. Therefore, the MFR therapist helps to resolve the reason the client was labelled with that condition, not the symptoms of the condition.

Some therapists new to MFR struggle to find resolution for their clients because they have not yet grasped the less-is-more approach or the whole-body approach. Once they grasp the concept of finding and following restrictions within the three-dimensional fascial network that can create pain anywhere in the body, their treatments rise to an entirely new level.

MFR Versus Other Massage Modalities

In treating the fascial complex, we influence not just the physicality of the tissue but also the emotions, memories and thoughts that are stored within each and every cell. The energy created within the personality ultimately influences our physicality. When we are upset or angry, that emotion is stored in the body. It may end up sitting in the equivalent of the body's waste bin, but it has to live somewhere. Wherever it does, it influences our actions and reactions just like a computer virus.

MFR should be viewed and utilised as an integrated approach, and its many unique characteristics make it completely different to massage. Some of these differentiating characteristics of the MFR approach described in this book include the following:

- Works on the entire fascial matrix and not only muscles or muscle lengths and their associated fascial sheaths
- Finds the pain and looks elsewhere for the cause
- Has a time element to allow the fascia to yield to touch without force in a three-dimensional manner
- Engages the client in the entire process, promoting communication to enhance the response to the treatment
- Encourages clients to allow their minds and bodies to soften, promoting inner awareness (interoception)
- Can, as a response to the treatment, involve a dynamic, spontaneous movement called unwinding
- Is not protocol or session-length orientated; each session offers a unique treatment
- Can be used as a home programme for rehabilitation and self-care approaches including fascial stretching
- Works not only with the physical but also the emotional responses to trauma
- With the integration of the MFR hands-on techniques, treats the pain as well as the emotional bracing and holding patterns that, left untreated, eventually create havoc in the system

Benefits of MFR

Following are some of the many benefits of MFR:

- General increase in health due to the increase in water volume (bound water) in the ground substance (nutrient and waste exchange)
- Promotion of relaxation and a sense of well-being
- Elimination of general pain and discomfort
- Increased proprioception and interoception
- Re-established and improved joint range of motion and muscle function

- Improved digestion, absorption and elimination
- Restored balance and promotion of correct posture
- Injury recovery and rehabilitation
- Can be used as part of an athletic or sport training routine and maintenance programme to promote mobility and performance
- Promotion of awareness of emotional issues and how they may be resolved

The benefits for therapists using MFR in their treatments are as follows:

- Is easy to learn and apply
- Can be easily integrated into existing practices
- Offers diversity in treatment approaches
- Increases career longevity because it is easy on the therapist's body and hands
- Increases a sense of touch and intuition

MFR Treatment Sessions

MFR should be carried out on clients as soon as possible after an injury to assist in the repair process and to avoid the knock-on effect of compensation. However, working in and around a scar site should be avoided for approximately six to eight weeks post-injury.

Not only can MFR attenuate fascial densification and fascial adhesions from scarring that may be contributing to pain, but it is also a relaxation tool for those who are post-surgery, postpartum or going through medical treatment. Therapists should always discuss MFR treatment with people in these situations and obtain their doctor's permission before commencing MFR therapy.

MFR can be undertaken as single sessions, usually an hour in length or longer based on the client's preference. Because MFR is a slow, gentle process, many clients benefit from two to three hours per session because this gives the therapist time to cover the entire body. This promotes total-body softening and yielding and offers the client a new position in space that is more energy efficient, flexible and pain free. The more regular the treatment sessions are, the more the client will benefit because the therapist can address the layers of restrictions and compensatory patterns as they appear. Clients benefit from an accumulation of MFR sessions as they begin to feel more freedom of movement and reduced tension.

MFR is also often offered as a multi-therapist treatment in which two or three therapists work together on one client. Multi-therapist treatments offer the client extra hands to get into positions that one pair of hands simply can't manage. This is discussed in more detail in chapter 13.

Normally, MFR is carried out in a clinic, treatment centre, hospital or healthcare practice. Many therapists work from home or travel to their clients' homes to practise. However, MFR can also be found in sports clubs and centres, private clinics, and dentists' and doctors' surgeries. Because MFR therapists do not need any tools, oils or lotions, and sometimes not even a treatment table, treatments can be done anywhere as long as the therapist can apply the techniques skin on skin with appropriate draping.

MFR offers a profound reduction of stored physical and emotional tension. For this reason, it is not advisable to use MFR for clients who have to perform tasks at optimal levels on the same day as a treatment. For example, a client who will be performing in a sporting competition or dance performance perhaps should not receive an MFR treatment on the same day. However, this can be negotiated with the client because people have unique needs. MFR can be applied to anyone at any age with the exception of those with the contraindications mentioned in chapter 3.

Closing Remarks

MFR is an individualised therapy approach that requires time for assessment and treatment. The body should never be forced. Take time with each technique offered in this book, listen to your hands and follow each unique perception of tissue change. Keep in mind, it's not how much pressure you use but how much resistance you feel.

Remembering the following basic concepts will help you use MFR to its full potential:

- Assess, palpate and treat the entire body.
- Always perform MFR skin on skin, never through clothing, towels or drapes. To avoid slipping on the skin, do not use massage oil, lotion or wax.
- Lean into the client with your hands, engage the tissue barrier (or end-feel) and do not force past it. Wait until you perceive a sense of tissue melting, and then take up the available tissue slack to the next barrier.
- Hold each technique for approximately three to five minutes or more to allow the physiological change within the tissues to take place.
- Do not allow your hands to slip or glide over the client's skin; this is massage, not MFR.
- Give the client permission to allow thoughts, feelings and memories to surface; never judge or lead the client in any way.

Quick Questions

1. In what ways is working with the three-dimensional fascial matrix different to working with muscles?
2. What is bound water?
3. What is another name for the superficial fascia?
4. How many seconds does it take for fascia to begin to respond to touch?
5. What are the three main constituents of fascia?

Initial Assessment

The initial assessment with the client is a very important part of any treatment. It is when you obtain all of the client's relevant personal and medical details as well as their symptoms and injury history. Don't forget the consent for treatment. Always welcome the client with a smile and make eye contact and shake hands if you feel that's appropriate. This will set you off on the right foot. Let the client get settled in your treatment room, and then begin your consultation process. You may prefer that the client complete the form prior to entering the room, or you may prefer to fill the form out with the client; either is acceptable.

The most important part of a consultation is listening to the client, who generally knows more about their symptoms and condition than you do. Many clients have attended a plethora of consultant appointments, outpatient appointments and physiotherapy sessions and have undergone scans, tests and X-rays and are still in pain. This is mostly because soft tissue injuries don't show up on regular tests and so can go undiagnosed, leading to further emotional issues for the client, not to mention the continual and consistent binding down of the tissue as time goes on, exacerbating the pain.

The physical assessment follows from obtaining the details in the consultation process. Physical assessments depend on the scope of practice. Not all therapists are trained in special orthopaedic tests or using measurement equipment such as a goniometer (a device for measuring angles of joint range, a bit like a specialised protractor). Physical assessments include postural evaluations, evaluations of available ranges of movement at the joints and palpation of the soft tissues. Some therapists also assess gait and perform specific muscle testing.

CLIENT TALK

Many of my clients who are in chronic pain feel that they have never been listened to when they discuss their symptoms and that they are nothing but statistics to practitioners. This is why it's really important that you listen to your clients, preferably without initially writing anything down, so that your focus is on them.

Client Consultation

Many clients come to MFR after trying a variety of other manual therapies, usually because they have been referred or have found information online or via word of mouth. Make sure to ask clients whether they have used other therapy approaches and what the results were. Any information is good information. This also gives you a clue about what they might be expecting, what they don't want and what they do want.

Set the scene right from the beginning by looking, watching and listening so that you can read between the lines. Always do the following:

- Welcome clients into the treatment room.
- Look at clients when they are talking, keep an open posture and be an active listener.
- Watch their body language and notice how they describe their symptoms.
- Notice the way they sit, stand and walk.
- Encourage them to describe their symptoms.

Doing all of the preceding helps boost the client's confidence in you as well as provides you with important information that will help you with your treatment. Take time to do the evaluation. It can take 30 to 40 minutes, less if the client completes the consultation form beforehand.

The consultation is not just about obtaining information; this is generally the time you are building rapport with your client. Having confidence in taking the history and being able to discuss medications, surgeries, pain patterns and pain history are important. Take time to discuss the information the client is offering. If you are unsure about medications, conditions and symptoms, ask the client; you are not expected to know everything. You can always check information about the condition online after the initial treatment.

Each therapy modality has its own style of medical intake and consultation form and objective assessments reflecting the scope of practice. A Swedish massage therapist's form may look quite different to that of a sports therapist, who is more likely to be dealing with chronic and acute injuries. MFR, because it is more of a remedial style of therapy, requires a closer look at the client's posture, including from a fascial point of view, as well as details about the client's pain history and information about any surgery, injuries and traumas.

The consultation form needs to be to the point and relative to the therapy and should elicit information that can be reassessed in subsequent sessions. In my practice, I try to use words other than *pain*. I want to acknowledge that clients are in pain, but I also want to help them lessen the burden of the pain by describing it in a less jarring way. Using the word *discomfort* is an option. A question such as, What's your primary reason for receiving treatment? works equally well. Like all other therapies, MFR requires a signature from the client providing permission to receive treatment.

The form should request the client's name, full address and contact information including home and mobile telephone numbers and email address. Ensure that you have gotten correct contact details in case you need to reschedule or cancel any appointments. It's also a good idea to know whether the client has been referred by someone because this provides marketing information and also gives you an indication of what the client might be expecting from the treatment. Obtain the name and contact information of the client's general practitioner (GP) in case of an emergency. This also enables you to write to the GP, with the client's permission, to report what the client presented with and how you were able to help. This demonstrates good communication skills and also allows you to do a bit of marketing too.

Figure 2.1, provided at the end of this chapter, is a sample form that prompts a patient to provide basic personal information, medical history, general health information and details about the reasons for receiving treatment. This form also includes a consent for treatment to be signed by the patient.

You need to learn to read between the lines with your clients. Sometimes what clients physically do or don't say provides more information than what they do say during the consultation process; this non-verbal communication can provide greater insight into clients' symptoms. Facial expressions, gestures and vocabulary may indicate how clients feel about their symptoms and condition and whether they actually believe that they can get better; all of this information can help you during the MFR session. How clients describe their symptoms and how they offer information can also signify their learning styles and personalities. You can use this information to help guide the descriptions of your treatment in a way that is more understandable and appropriate to their needs—we call this mirroring.

In an MFR treatment consultation you should do the following:

- Obtain client information and a medical consultation form.
- Read back and confirm what the client has written.
- Discuss the client's symptoms, onset and progression, treatment and tests.
- Ask about medication.
- Ask about any dental treatment and any previous surgeries.
- Ask about any injuries, falls and car accidents.

Up until this point the client should remain clothed or at least in a treatment gown, if you use them. Many clients are desperate to get their clothes off to get on the treatment table as soon as possible. It's polite and professional to tell them what form the session will take as soon as they enter the room to make them feel as comfortable as possible about the entire session.

This form includes patient intake and medical history information, as well as consent to receive treatment.

Your Personal Details

Today's date _____

Name _____ Date of birth _____ Age _____

Address _____ Occupation _____

General practitioner (GP) contact details _____

Post code _____

Telephone number _____ Mobile number _____

Email address _____ How referred _____

Medical History (Include Dates)

Surgeries and procedures: _____

_____

_____

Fractures: _____

_____

_____

Accidents: _____

_____

_____

Current medications (prescription and over the counter) and alternative supplements:

_____

_____

_____

Have you been referred for further investigation, outpatient therapy, physiotherapy or other therapy by your general practitioner? If so, for what and when? _____

_____

_____

_____

Figure 2.1   Sample form for a patient to fill out providing basic personal information, medical history, general health information and details about the reasons for receiving treatment.

Figure 2.1   > *continued*

Health Problems

Do you have, or have you ever had, any of the following conditions? (Tick all that apply.)

☐ circulatory disorder

☐ respiratory disorder

☐ COVID-19

☐ heart condition

☐ high or low
  blood pressure

☐ thrombosis

☐ dizziness

☐ blackouts

☐ dental complaints

☐ varicose veins

☐ epilepsy

☐ diabetes

☐ abdominal complaints

☐ skin disorder

☐ bowel complaints

☐ bladder complaints

☐ visual disturbance

☐ allergies

☐ arthritis

☐ osteoporosis or
  osteopenia

☐ nervous system
  disorder (MS, stroke)

☐ headaches

☐ tinnitus (ringing
  in the ears)

☐ eating disorder

☐ a potentially fatal
  condition

General

Height _____ Weight _____ Special diet_____

Smoker?   Yes   No   If yes, how many per day? _____

How much water do you drink? _____ /day

Alcohol consumption   light   moderate   heavy

Sport, exercise and relaxation: _____

_____

_____

How would you describe your stress levels?   high   moderate   low

Your Reasons for Treatment

What are your expectations of this treatment?_____

_____

_____

Primary Reason for Receiving Treatment

What is your primary complaint? _____

_____

_____

When and how did this complaint start? _____

_____

_____

Figure 2.1   *> continued*

How does this complaint affect you? _____

_____

_____

Is this a recurrence of an old injury?   yes   no

If yes, when did the old injury occur? _____

Indicate your current level of discomfort (10 is the worst and 0 is the least):

0   1   2   3   4   5   6   7   8   9   10

Indicate the worst level of intensity you have had with your primary complaint (10 is the worst and 0 is the least):

0   1   2   3   4   5   6   7   8   9   10

When did the worst level of intensity occur? _____

_____

What, if anything, increases your pain and discomfort? _____

_____

What, if anything, decreases your pain or discomfort? _____

_____

How often does your pain or discomfort occur on a normal day? (10 is constant and 0 is never.)

0   1   2   3   4   5   6   7   8   9   10
Never   Constant

At what time of day is your pain or discomfort at its worst? (Circle those that apply.)

on waking   midday   evening   before bed   during the night

To what extent (percentage) is your daily functional ability hindered as the result of your pain or discomfort? (Circle where 0% is the worst and 100% is the best.)

On a good day: 0%   10%   20%   30%   40%   50%   60%   70%   80%   90%   100%

On a bad day: 0%   10%   20%   30%   40%   50%   60%   70%   80%   90%   100%

Have you had any previous treatment for this complaint? If so, what was it and what was the outcome? _____

_____

_____

Have you had any X-rays, tests or MRIs? If so, what were the results?   yes   no

_____

_____

Figure 2.1   *> continued*

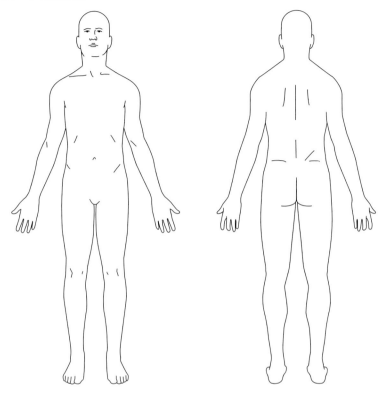

Shade on the diagram the areas where you feel your pain or discomfort. Mark on the diagram with a cross (x) where you feel areas of numbness or tingling.

If you are employed, how many days have you been absent from work for this pain or discomfort? _____

Indicate any other information that you think is relevant to your symptoms and treatment of your primary complaint. _____

_____

_____

Other Reasons for Receiving Treatment

Do you have any additional reasons for seeking treatment? _____

_____

_____

_____

Figure 2.1 *> continued*

Summarise any previous or ongoing treatments or physician referrals for your secondary complaint, including appropriate dates and outcomes. _____

_____

_____

_____

Indicate any other information that you think is relevant to your symptoms and treatment of your secondary complaint. _____

_____

_____

_____

Have you at any time had treatment for a dental or jaw issue including wearing a mouth guard, braces, dental bridge or dentures? _____

_____

_____

_____

Have you at any time been prescribed orthotics, heel lifts, or arch supports or had any treatment for foot and ankle issues? _____

_____

_____

_____

Consent for Treatment and Physical Examination

Thank you for providing us with information on your medical status and your personal details. An MFR treatment consists of a discussion concerning general medical information and specific information regarding your present complaint, after which a physical examination will be carried out. This will include an in-depth assessment of your presenting complaint as well as any other relevant examination procedures. You will be required to change down to your underwear, or if you prefer, shorts and a bra top. During treatment you will be draped with sheets or towels.

On subsequent treatments, further assessments will be carried out to establish changes to your posture, function and presenting complaint.

Children will not be treated without a parent or guardian's permission.

Signature of client _____ Date _____

Signature of therapist _____ Date _____

Medical History

A medical history provides details of any surgeries, fractures, accidents or injuries your clients have had. You also need to know about any medications they are currently taking, including prescriptive and over-the-counter medications as well as supplements, vitamins, minerals and herbal medications. If a client is on medication for a condition that is not a contraindication for MFR, all you need to know is the amount of medication taken and when it is taken. If you are unfamiliar with some of the medications, ask the client what they are, what they do and how long the client has been on them, and consider whether they are contraindicated for MFR. You can buy a medications dictionary and index book, which provide all of the information you need about medications. You also can call the client's GP for more information or search on the internet.

You also need to know whether a client is still under investigation for any conditions and discomfort through a GP, outpatient clinic, consultant or physiotherapy or pain clinic. You will need to decide whether the current condition contraindicates MFR treatment from you. I would be more concerned about offering treatment to someone who wants MFR for abdominal discomfort and who is still under referral to a gastrointestinal consultant than about someone who has been through the

Effective Questioning

Effective questioning involves asking questions that require full descriptive answers. Closed questions, to which the answer is either yes or no, might look like this:

- Have you talked to your doctor about your symptoms?
- Does your discomfort keep you from sleeping?
- Does your discomfort last all day?

Effective questioning involves asking open-ended questions that require more than a yes or no answer. Such questions engage the client in conversation and provide more information. Many clients have seen many specialists who have not been able to diagnose or even understand their symptoms. They may feel that they have never been listened to and have been passed from pillar to post. Open-ended questions allow you to make clients feel confident that you are interested in them and not just in relieving their discomfort. You want them to know that they are not a label, a condition or a statistic but a person who needs your time, empathy and understanding.

Following are some examples of open-ended questions:

- How would you describe your symptoms?
- How did the consultation go with the specialist?
- How are your symptoms affecting you?
- How did your symptoms start?

entire process from GP to consultant and is now attending pain clinics because no one can find any cause of the pain. Such information should be covered when the client books an appointment, so you don't waste your time or his.

MFR will enhance the efficacy of other manual therapy treatments the client may be receiving, such as physiotherapy, osteopathy and chiropractic. The only problem with combining therapies is that you will not have a clear indication of what is and is not working. Some therapists prefer that soft tissue therapies be performed before manual osseous adjustments so that the tissue is soft enough to receive the adjustments and will hold them for a longer period of time.

CLIENT TALK

I always tell my clients that if they have a therapy they enjoy and receive benefit from, such as acupuncture, massage or energy work, they should keep receiving those treatments to enhance their relaxation process. I let them know that these therapies help each other as well as enhance their MFR treatments.

The consultation form lists conditions and asks the client to acknowledge whether they have ever suffered from them; these include congenital (inherited) and contracted conditions followed by the primary, and possibly secondary, reason for wanting to receive MFR. The primary condition is the reason the client is looking to receive MFR therapy. You need to know the following:

- What the symptom is
- When it started
- How it started
- Whether it is a recurrence of an old injury or pain
- How it affects the client
- What it stops the client from doing
- What makes the symptom better
- What makes the symptom worse

Take time to discuss all of the client's symptoms and ask for a description of the discomfort and whether it changes during the day.

Because most clients receiving MFR have chronic conditions and discomfort, an orthopaedic physical assessment pain scale, in which the number 1 refers to the least amount of pain and the number 10 refers to the most, can be very helpful. Pain scales help clients describe their current level of discomfort, when it is at its worst and how often it affects them on a normal day. You can also add questions about the level of their discomfort on a good day and on a bad day. Some therapists like to include a body diagram so clients can indicate where their discomfort is and identify areas of tension, numbness or tingling. Form 2.1, provided earlier in this chapter, includes such a diagram. You would then have one body chart with subjective information and another (your postural evaluation, discussed later) with objective information.

You also need to know whether your client has had any tests, scans or X-rays and whether they were inconclusive, as well as any treatment the client has had through their healthcare provider, what that treatment was and whether it was beneficial. The form should include some space where the client can fill in any other information about why they are seeking treatment. See form 2.1 at the end of this chapter for some examples. Give them the opportunity to offer information that may not be addressed in other forms of treatment.

For example, the client may believe that food intolerances and allergies are related to their symptoms or that emotional issues, work-related issues, stress or a difficult childbirth may be relevant.

TIP Make sure the client signs and dates the medical history form, and offer to provide a copy if required. Some therapy training providers and members of professional associations also require the signature of the therapist performing the consultation and subsequent assessment and treatment; check with your own professional association for guidance.

Some clients are so desperate to get on with the treatment that they fail to fill in the initial consultation form adequately and accurately. To protect you and your client, go through the form together, diligently making sure you have the information you need to progress with the treatment.

Key Follow-Up Questions

You may wish to consider the following items because they will have a direct impact on your client's function and may be influencing, or even causing, the dysfunction and discomfort.

- Ask the client what their job is and whether they have to stay standing or seated all day with little or no opportunity to move around. Do they use a computer or drive all day? What they do for a living will have a direct impact on what you see in the postural evaluation.

- Note whether the client uses a computer mouse at a computer or works from a laptop on their knees. Clients who sit all day normally present with an anterior pelvic tilt and may complain of low back discomfort.

- Another key factor to low back issues and pelvic imbalances are repetitively sitting with the legs crossed or sitting for long periods of time with a wallet or mobile phone in a back pocket. These positions mechanically perpetuate a pelvic imbalance resulting in dysfunction and discomfort.

- Other factors include new running shoes or continually wearing old shoes that lack arch support, including ill-fitting slippers.

> continued

> continued

- Sleeping position is also a consideration because continually being in one position will affect the back, shoulders and neck, particularly if that position is on the abdomen or with the arms overhead.

- You also need to know whether the client regularly plays a sport or goes to the gym and what their hobbies are. Repetitive strain injuries will also present in the postural assessment and may be causing the discomfort.

- Make sure to ask the client if they have ever had any problems with their jaw or wear a mouth guard. Most clients don't realise that a relationship exists between tension in the jaw and the tension and discomfort in the rest of the body.

- Ask whether the client wears any kind of insoles or heel lifts in their shoes. If they wear heel lifts, ask for as much information as possible. Were the heel lifts specially made or purchased over the counter? What was the reason for getting them in the first place? Clients are given foot orthotics not just for foot and ankle pain and discomfort but for back issues, pelvic imbalances, leg length discrepancies and even jaw pain. If you perform MFR on clients who regularly wear orthotics, you may not be able to provide lasting relief from the symptoms until you work with the reason they got the orthotics in the first place. There is no use spending lots of time using MFR to balance the body when as soon as the client puts their shoes back on, they knock it all out of place again.

- If your client is wearing orthotics for pain and discomfort, work with them and the specialist who prescribed them to eventually get to the stage where the orthotics are no longer needed. Explain to the client that using heel lifts can perpetuate a leg length and pelvic imbalance and that your goal through MFR is to balance the entire body so that orthotics are no longer needed. Always do this process slowly and gradually with the consent and understanding of any other healthcare specialist involved.

Physical Assessment

The physical assessment is performed after the initial questioning and completion of the client medical and personal details form and is split into two parts: with the client standing (postural assessment including a visual and palpatory assessment) and with the client on the treatment table (palpatory assessment). The palpatory assessments will be discussed in chapter 4. You should obtain a signature of consent from the client permitting you to perform a physical postural and palpatory assessment.

A postural visual assessment offers a good indication of the client's degree of balance and imbalance. At the very least, you should notice what looks balanced and what doesn't and then perform some techniques and have a look again to see what has changed. Performing a postural assessment and palpation evaluation at the beginning and sometimes the end of the session as well will enhance your treatment and help both you and your client observe the progression of the client's response to the treatment.

What the functional evaluation includes depends on the treatment modality. Most physiotherapists, chiropractors, osteopaths and sports and remedial massage therapists routinely screen for joint and muscle range, whereas holistic and relaxation massage therapists may not. The important thing is to conduct an adequate evaluation both before and after treatment to determine treatment progression and help the client observe any changes from the treatment.

An MFR treatment session may include any or all of the following:

- Standing visual postural assessment followed by a palpatory assessment
- Movement and gait analysis
- Orthopaedic assessment and special tests
- Goniometer measurements (a tool used to measure angles of range of movement)
- Postural photographs (with client permission only)

The physical assessment can include a variety of assessment methods depending on your scope of practice. At each session, ask the client about any responses from the last treatment and any present symptoms. This book describes the assessment tools of postural evaluation (later in this chapter) and palpation (discussed in chapter 4). Specific testing for joint ranges and gait assessment requires special training and thus is beyond the scope of this book.

TIP
- Ask the client to provide the details of all injuries, accidents and surgical interventions because the fascial system stores a lifetime of injurious events that continually affect function and form.
- Ask your clients not to wear body moisturiser or fake tanning products on the day of the treatment because these products may cause your hands to slip on the skin.
- Clients are generally treated in their underwear; however, some clients may prefer to wear loose-fitting shorts and a vest top.
- Front-fastening and sport bras make performing MFR on the client's back challenging. Ask the client if she is willing to remove her bra and drape her accordingly, and ask her to wear an alternative for subsequent treatments.
- Because MFR is always performed skin on skin, some techniques may require you to slip your hands under bra straps and the edges of underwear. Always ask permission to do this. If you believe it is necessary, add a reference to this in the consent portion of your consultation form.

Postural Evaluation

The most important thing to look for in a postural evaluation is equality and balance. It is not about diagnosing the client's discomfort. There are so many ways to look at the human body and make sense of dysfunction. If one leg is more externally rotated than the other, logic would make us look at the external hip rotator muscles. However, the leg may have to rotate externally because of a pelvic imbalance and low back dysfunction, which may be the result of a car crash 10 years ago. The easiest way to perform a postural evaluation is to identify what looks balanced and what doesn't.

You also have to take into consideration that when standing, the client may be in a compensational habitual holding pattern from an old injury or from a repetitive strain pattern from sport, work or even a sleeping position. What you see may be contributing to the current dysfunction and discomfort, but it may also be covering up something deeper that may have been inadequately treated or in some cases never treated at all.

In standing, the body is working against gravity and organising itself in a position that is the most efficient and pain free. No one stands all day, and the client's pain may not even occur whilst standing. When you look for what is balanced and imbalanced before you treat the client, you can then see the changes you make by re-evaluating both during and after treatment. No one's body is perfectly balanced, nor does it need to be. Your goal is to help the client return to a pain-free, active lifestyle.

How you perform a postural and palpatory assessment is up to you. The important thing is that you have a process that you can use to compare your initial assessment with later assessments as treatment progresses. As in all palpatory assessments and techniques, make sure to use soft and gentle hands if you need to touch the client's body. Set the intention to make a connection with your client by effectively communicating.

Following are the steps of a visual postural assessment:

1. Ask your client to remove their clothing with exception of their underwear, including socks. In all postural evaluations, you have to be able to see and feel as much of the skin as possible. If the client is not comfortable standing in their underwear, shorts or swimwear (a two-piece bathing suit for women) is acceptable.

2. If your client has long hair, ask them to tie it up so you can see and feel around their neck and skull. I have a bag of spare hair bands in a drawer in my treatment room for clients who don't have them.

3. Ask the client to stand in a natural standing position. Many clients try to adopt their best posture—tall and upright. Unfortunately, this forces the body into an unnatural posture. Suggest that the client relax and stand in the most normal position possible.

4. Look first for balance and symmetry from the front, back and both sides, writing down what you see.

CLIENT TALK

Even though clients understand the process of postural evaluation, no one likes being stared at, particularly when wearing just underwear. Try to make the client feel at ease by talking, and always keep your treatment room warm.

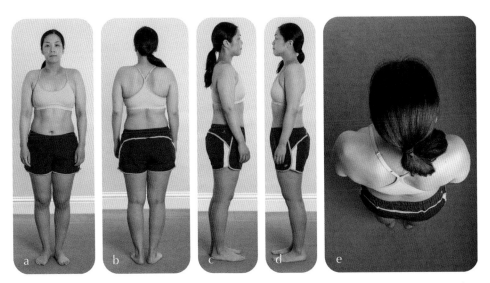

Figure 2.2   Positions from which to view the body are (a) anterior, (b) posterior, (c-d) lateral and (e) transverse.

Following are five positions from which to view the body (see figure 2.2):

- Front (anterior) view
- Back (posterior) view
- Right side (lateral) view
- Left side (lateral) view
- From the top down (transverse view)

The two plumb lines in the body indicate balance in the anterior and posterior views from right to left and also indicate balance in the centre of gravity (COG) in the right and left lateral views. The central plumb line on the anterior and posterior views should completely bisect the body down the middle and runs from between the feet, through the pubic symphysis, navel, sternum, manubrium, middle of the chin, nose, between the eyes to the crown of the head and, correspondingly, from between the feet through the coccyx and straight up the spine to the top of the head. The lateral plumb line runs from the anterior aspect of the lateral malleoli through the knee, the greater trochanter, the middle of the lumbar vertebrae, the acromion process, the middle of the cervical vertebrae and through the ear to the top of the head.

Anterior View Posture Questions

- Are the big toes equal, rolling in or out or shifting?
- Are the feet falling or rolling in or out?
- Are the ankles and feet externally or internally rotated?
- Are the kneecaps pointing forwards or to the side?
- Are the legs knock-kneed, bowlegged or straight?

- Is the muscle tone the same on both legs?
- Are the anterior superior iliac spines (ASIS) and pelvic rims level?
- Does the thorax sit level on top of the pelvis?
- Is the belly button in the middle of the abdomen or pulled to the side?
- Are the arches or angles of the ribs level?
- Is the pectoralis, or breast area, level?
- Are the sternoclavicular (SC) joints level?
- Is the distance from the cervical spine to the acromion process the same on the right and left sides?
- Does the shoulder girdle sit level on top of the thorax and pelvis?
- Are the ears level?
- Is the head tilted or side bent or rotated on the cervical spine?
- Are the arms level by the sides of the body?
- Do the arms rotate in or out?
- Is the space between the arm and the body the same on both sides?
- Are the eyes level?
- Is the jaw level?
- Is the nose central or pulled to the side?

Posterior View Posture Questions

- Are the feet falling or rolling in or out?
- Are the ankles and feet externally or internally rotated?
- Are the Achilles tendons level?
- Are the calf muscles equal?
- Are the creases at the back of the knees equal?
- Are the legs knock-kneed, bowlegged or straight?
- Are the legs equal underneath the pelvis or over the feet?
- Are the gluteal folds equal?
- Are the posterior superior iliac spines (PSIS) and pelvic rims equal?
- Does the thorax sit level on top of the pelvis?
- Are the folds of skin in the back (or legs) equal?
- Are the scapula equal or winged?
- Is the space between the body and arm equal on both sides?
- Do the arms rotate in or out?
- Are the arms level by the sides of the body?
- Is the distance from the cervical spine to the acromion process the same on the right and left sides?
- Does the shoulder girdle sit level on top of the thorax and pelvis?

- Are the ears level?
- Is the head tilted or side bent or rotated on the cervical spine?

Lateral View Posture Questions

- Do some parts of the body lie more in front or behind the plumb line in general?
- Do the knees hyperextend or stay more flexed?
- Do the hips fall in front of the plumb line or behind?
- Are the PSIS and ASIS level on the same horizontal plane? (In women the ASIS is usually slightly lower than the PSIS.)
- Which parts of the spine are more in front of or behind the plumb line?
- Is the head protracted or retracted?
- Is the cervical spine flat or curved?
- Is the head tilted backwards?
- Are both sides the same?

The transverse plane is easiest to look at by standing close behind the client. Tell the client what you are going to do, and then look straight down their back to see if the hips stack equally on the legs, the thorax on the hips, shoulders on the thorax and head on the shoulders (see figure 2.3). Stand on a stool if you need to so you can clearly determine the degree of balance (or lack thereof).

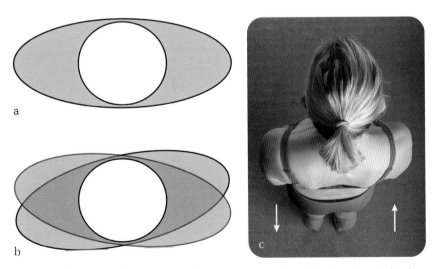

Figure 2.3 Postural assessment of the transverse plane. The head and shoulders should be in line with each other (a), and the shoulders evenly stacked on the thorax, hips and so on. If the transverse plane is imbalanced, the shoulders may be rotated relative to the head (b). (c) This person shows an imbalance of the hips on the legs and the thorax on the hips. The right-hand side of the body is more anterior than the left side; the right side of the body is rotating to the left.

Doing this gives you a clue about rotations in relationship to what you saw in the lateral views. If you see in the right lateral view that the upper body is more anterior of the plumb line than it was from the left lateral view, then in the transverse plane you should see the body rotating to the left when you look down the back.

If you are confident about performing a postural evaluation, you may want to include other factors to help you distinguish balance from imbalance. If you are not very confident about performing the postural evaluation, use only five or six landmarks from each of the four views and mark them on your postural assessment chart. The landmarks I use are the ankle bones; the knees; the ASIS from the front and the PSIS from the back; the inferior angles of the scapulae from the back; and the SC joints from the front, the shoulders and the ears. From the lateral views I look at the ankles, knees, pelvis, thorax and ears.

Chart Notation

If you and other therapists are treating the same clients, you will want to use the same terms and shorthand to ensure that you understand each other's notes. Start by drawing lines on your body charts for structural symmetry and asymmetry. If you see one shoulder higher than the other in the anterior view, draw a line between those two points at an angle representing which shoulder is higher. Do the same for all the other points you have chosen on the anterior and posterior views.

On the lateral views, draw arrows to indicate where the client's body is in front of or behind the lateral plumb line. Shade in or put Xs on areas of pain and tension unless you already have this as a subjective assessment on your consultation form from the client. Take as many notes as you can or, even better, take photographs (with permission).

Add all of what you see to the information provided by the client to get a better idea of the pain and dysfunction. This comprehensive postural assessment will help in the treatment as well as the post-treatment reassessment in which you perform the same postural assessment that you did initially. This provides an indication of what has changed, softened and balanced and also helps you decide where to treat next.

Foot and Leg Observations

Look at the client's feet and legs from the anterior and posterior views. Drop an imaginary plumb line from the pubic symphysis to the floor between the feet. Imagine two right-angle triangles, back to back, between the legs. One side of the triangle is the plumb line, one side is the leg and one side is the floor. Is one triangle narrower than the other? The narrower triangle is usually on the side of the body where the leg is carrying most of the body weight. You can ask the client which leg carries most of the weight. Some will be able to tell you and some won't. You can draw this triangle in the corner of your postural assessment form and use it for a re-evaluation later.

Gravitational force flows through the spine onto the sacral base, where it is then distributed evenly through each acetabulum, right and left, down through the femur, the tibia and into the ankle and the calcaneus. Conversely, the body's anti-gravity system (the fascial matrix) pushes into the ground to stabilise the body, creating a counterforce that travels along the same pathway in the body superiorly. In response to abnormal pulls, strain patterns, tension and pain, the body tries to offer the best adaptation of normal it can in the most efficient and pain-free manner. This may result in the body weight being distributed unevenly. When that posture becomes exhausted, the body slowly creeps into another position in space that can support the tension imposed on it. Eventually, the demands become too much resulting in pain and dysfunction.

The problem is never as simple as a fallen arch, an anteriorly rotated hip, a lateral side bend of the lumbar vertebrae or a winged scapula. The body is a totally uninterrupted and integrated system from top to toe because the fascial system connects all the bones, muscles, nerves and vessels. If the legs are not balanced and the body weight is not supported evenly on them, then everything above won't have a firm foundation and will then have to compensate to function.

Pelvic Observations

In chapter 4, we discuss pelvic observations further and perform a palpatory assessment of the bony landmarks of the pelvis, namely the ASIS and the PSIS. This discussion offers information regarding balance and function of the middle of the body and therefore provides a greater insight into system-wide dysfunction. When these points are not on the same horizontal plane, imbalance also occurs within the pelvic bowl, creating a myriad of internal symptoms as its contents become crushed and twisted (not to mention complications in childbirth). Some studies state that the ASIS should be slightly lower than the PSIS on the same side (i.e., a slight anterior pelvic tilt), particularly in women. However, if you find a difference in height between the two ASIS from an anterior view, this means that one side of the pelvis is tilted more anteriorly than its counterpart. This indicates a pelvic imbalance.

Jaw Observations

Lastly, let's look at the jaw. The jaw is the only bilateral jointed bone in the body. It has a synovial joint on either side of the head, which has an articular disc. Any imbalance and dysfunction in the human body will always be represented in the jaw, and vice versa. It is very common for clients suffering pelvic dysfunction and back pain to have a history of jaw issues; some wear night splints or braces.

Some clients complain of a clicking and popping jaw that no number of visits to the dentist have resolved. A look at the relationship between the fascial network and the osseous spacers in the tensegrity model makes clear that balance must be created in the entire structure below the jaw to resolve its pain and dysfunction.

Practical Application: Pelvic Dysfunctions

This practical test with clients helps them understand why we work with the body as a whole by illustrating how the pelvis moves and how dysfunction can exist. Guide the patient through these steps.

1. Stand up and place your hands on your hip bones over both your ASIS.

2. Make sure your feet are equally beneath your hips and are pointing forwards.

3. Without moving your feet, rotate your hips and body to the left.

4. Notice how the right side of your pelvis begins to tilt anteriorly, forwards and down, whilst the left side of your pelvis tilts posteriorly, backwards and up.

5. What do you notice happening in your legs? Your right leg will begin to medially, or internally, rotate, and your left leg will begin to laterally, or externally, rotate at the same time.

6. Now feel your knees; your right knee bends whilst your left knee extends.

7. Now feel your feet; your right medial arch has fallen and your body weight is on the inside of that foot and on the outside of the left foot.

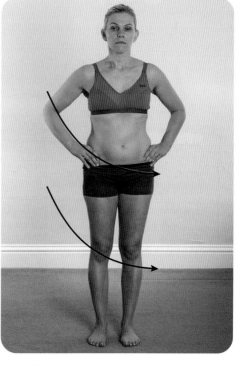

You can now see how feet and knee issues can be caused when the pelvis is out of balance and that foot issues can create low back symptoms because the pelvis supporting the spine isn't supported evenly from below.

Practical Application: Functional Imbalance

Every person has a dominant side; the side on which they sleep, use more for work or to play sport and for compensation against pain and dysfunction. Following is an easy way to understand how a shorter and tighter lateral side of the body affects the entire system.

1. In standing, pull your hips and ribs closer together on the right side of your body without lifting your foot off the floor.

2. When you shorten the lateral side, the opposite shoulder lifts superiorly. What you are doing is laterally side bending your lumbar spine and shortening that side. The neck then side bends toward the lifted shoulder, creating tension and strain, a pelvic, thoracic and shoulder girdle imbalance and ultimately pain. If you have a shortening anywhere in your body, it will create various imbalances throughout the entire structure.

3. Most people have some kind of cervical imbalance, the most common of which is called a head-forward posture, where the head sits anteriorly over the thorax generating an abnormal pull of the tissues to stabilise and support it. When the cervical spine is compromised, correct shoulder function is greatly diminished due to the relationship between the osseous and soft tissue structures.

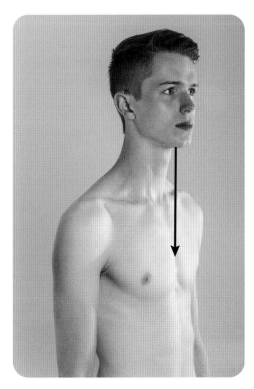

4. If we drop a plumb line from the chin, it should meet the manubrium at the top of the sternum, as shown in the photo. In most cases it meets the sternum about 0.7 inches (2 cm) farther down. Anything past the manubrium is technically a head-forward posture.

5. Now, in standing, pull your chin back and straighten your cervical spine.

6. In that position, raise both your arms into abduction to the sides of your body and up over your head as in a scapula glide test.

7. Feel how easy it is to raise your arms.

8. Now relax your neck and chin and jut your chin forwards, adopting a head-forward posture.

9. Now abduct your arms again up over your head. It's not as easy, is it?

To resolve shoulder issues, you must balance the thoracic and cervical spine on each other and on the pelvis, legs and feet.

Practical Application: Fascial Drag

Before finishing your postural assessment, you should look at fascial drag, which is when the tissues are being pulled, dragged and twisted as a result of tensional forces. It often can be clearly seen in clients' posture.

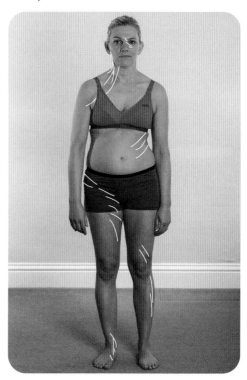

1. Stand a little farther back from your client, soften your focus and look at the body as a whole.

2. Imagine the pelvis as a cup. Is the cup spilling over anywhere or being dragged to one side more than the other?

3. Do you notice that the skin and underlying tissue is being pulled in one direction making it look as though the client has a dominant side?

4. Do you see a drag or pull through the ribcage, chest, neck and up into the face and jaw making it look as though one side of the face is longer than the other or one eye is lower than the other? This is fascial drag, and it occurs as a result of system-wide dysfunction and imbalance as a result of trauma, poor posture or inflammation.

5. With a contrasting-colour pen or pencil, shade in or draw lines on your body chart where you see fascial drag.

As with the rest of your postural assessment, re-evaluate any fascial drag post-treatment.

TIP
- Be diligent with your postural evaluations. The more you do them, the more you will learn and the more you will understand what to look and feel for.
- Share your information with your clients. This will help them understand the process of the treatment as well as offer insight into the progression with the treatment.
- Reassess at various times throughout treatment using the pain scales you used during the initial consultation. This will give you and the client an ongoing indication of treatment success.

Closing Remarks

When any structure is not level, tensional lines occur to maintain the strain pattern, which ultimately increases the imbalance. Eventually, some of the tissues become chronically short and some areas become taut and overstrained, thickening down in response to the oppositional pull. This is what causes pain, so even though a client may present with carpal tunnel syndrome, a frozen shoulder or lumbar pain, you have to ask yourself why. MFR is not a symptomatic treatment because you don't focus on the site of pain. Rather, you identify the pain and look and feel elsewhere in the body for tensional strain patterns that may be causing it.

Postural assessment can differ dramatically from one therapy modality to the next. Some therapists don't assess in standing at all but perform all their assessments on the treatment table. Most often the protocol for assessment involves logically looking and feeling for a model of specific items, analysing them and then using specific techniques to address them. This approach simply does not work for everyone, and if you have the mindset that you will find an issue, you will (even if it's not there). It is therefore prudent to take your time with evaluation and treat every person as unique. Like everything else, a postural evaluation takes time and improves with experience. Even if you are already proficient in postural assessment, try looking at your evaluation from a fascial point of view, looking for fascial drag, pulls and tensional lines that are creating imbalance. Always treat the person, not the symptom.

Always follow your postural assessment with a palpatory assessment (discussed in chapter 4) and describe to the client what you are looking and feeling for. The entire consultation process through to the end of the treatment session should be fluid, reflecting your confidence and care so the client feels at ease with the process and confident in your ability to help.

Where to start your treatment is the next question. Being able to note what you see is an essential tool but not much good if you don't know what to do with it. An easy approach is to start and treat the site of pain, then re-evaluate after performing a few techniques to see what has changed. However, be careful not to focus on the site of pain but to treat the entire body because no one part moves in isolation (tensegrity). Find the pain and look elsewhere for the cause. Or, start at the place where you believe you will make the biggest change in the structure, and after performing a few techniques re-evaluate and follow on from there.

Quick Questions

1. Why is listening to clients important?
2. Can sitting on a wallet or phone in a back pocket create an imbalance in the pelvis?
3. What are the five views to use when performing a postural assessment?
4. Do you need clients' signed permission to treat them?
5. What is the only bilateral jointed bone in the body?

Preparation and Communication

Because MFR is a hands-on therapy, it carries similar contraindications and treatment guidelines as general massage with only a few differences. Besides the consultation form and the evaluation process, a few other elements need to be addressed prior to treatment, including how MFR is performed. Contraindications must always be considered. And you need to always ask, Is this client suitable for MFR?

As with every other form of therapy, how you set up your treatment room and perform your treatments does not just promote you professionally but also determines longevity in your career. It is also important that you make clients feel comfortable throughout the process and that you adequately discuss their reasons for treatment as well as their responses to the treatment. This builds your confidence and your clients' confidence in you.

Contraindications

MFR is generally not a core qualification; basic soft tissue and fascial skills are often included in courses such as sports therapy and physiotherapy. Because MFR is generally a postgraduate remedial rehabilitation approach used by a variety of therapists, an understanding of pathology and contraindications is often already in place. Contraindications have to be in line with core training. For example, a physiotherapist using MFR would be able to work with a few more clients on the contraindications list than a massage therapist would. Check with your professional association if you need further clarification on this.

If a client presents with symptoms indicating the possibility of an underlying pathological state, or if you have any doubt, treat it as a contraindication and refer them to their doctor unless you are qualified to treat the condition. First, do no harm.

Following are lists of contraindications for the use of MFR, both global and local. In the case of local contraindications, you can work on the client, but stay clear of contraindicated areas.

Global Contraindications

- Alcohol and recreational drug use
- Febrile state (high temperature)
- Systemic infection
- Colds and flus that are contagious
- Acute circulatory conditions and acute blood disorders
- Deep vein thrombosis and aneurism
- Uncontrolled hypertension usually involving anti-coagulant therapy
- Severe undiagnosed swelling
- Severe undiagnosed pain
- Undiagnosed lumps
- Rapid weight loss or gain
- Undiagnosed breathing difficulties
- Undiagnosed bowel and bladder issues

Local Contraindications

- Open wounds
- Sutures or stitches
- Healing fracture
- Skin hypersensitivity or inflammation
- Infectious skin condition or sunburn
- Radiation therapy
- Localised infection
- Cortisone therapy (wait three or four days on the specific area)
- Osteomyelitis (avoid the inflamed areas; do not treat if the client has other systemic symptoms)
- Osteoporosis or advanced degenerative changes (avoid affected areas)
- Rheumatological conditions (avoid inflamed areas)
- Severe varicose veins

During MFR treatments, clients need to be able to note and describe what they are feeling. Clients on medications that dull the senses, such as anti-depressants, may need a little more time and help in responding to the therapy. Taking anti-depressants doesn't necessarily mean that the client has depression; these drugs are also used to treat other conditions such as chronic pain and insomnia. Be sure to ask your clients their reasons for being on medications, and take that into consideration during therapy.

How many times do clients turn up sick with a cold? Turning them away results in lost revenue, but working with them is a contraindication, not just for the client (because it can increase the infection), but for you. If you catch the cold from the client, you won't be able to work and you may pass it to other clients too. Consider posting on your website or brochures a request that clients not attend appointments when their temperatures are higher than normal, or they have a cold, flu or stomach bug. Explain the importance of keeping your treatment room free of germs.

Conversely, if you have a contagious infection, cold or flu, you shouldn't be treating clients. Apart from issues of contagion, it's simply not professional to be sniffing and coughing your way through treatments. You may need to take a few days off so you can recover and not pass on germs to your clients.

Three contraindications for MFR that are particularly important to mention are pregnancy, scar tissue and adhesions, and cancer (malignant tumours that are being treated with chemotherapy or radiotherapy, or that are in remission).

Pregnancy

MFR is an appropriate therapy for pregnant woman after their first trimester and can be extremely beneficial in preparation for labour. MFR helps to alleviate the stressful symptoms of body change and adaptation not only as the baby grows but as a result of the hormone relaxin being secreted into the system. Relaxin softens the cartilage at the pubic symphysis and the joints at the sacroiliac in preparation for labour. Many women suffer back and pelvic discomfort in these areas during pregnancy, and MFR can be an effective therapy to maintain the integrity of these areas. As with all other forms of bodywork, abdominal work is contraindicated during the entire pregnancy.

Some professional associations and therapy insurers permit practitioners to treat pregnant women without having to attend a pregnancy massage course; others require such courses. Be sure to check the guidelines of your professional association before accepting pregnant clients.

CLIENT TALK

Care and consideration are needed when working with clients with neurological, muscular spasm and spasticity conditions. These clients may require additional support and stability-orientated therapy and re-education to receive the maximum benefits from MFR.

I have treated a few clients with multiple sclerosis (MS) who have benefitted from MFR as a total-body approach; it has helped them to walk and balance with less effort.

Scar Tissue and Adhesions

Working with scars and adhesions is very rewarding because the benefits to the client are enormous. Not only are you making the scar look much softer and less angry, but you are attenuating potential restrictions that may be placed on vessels, nerves and organs. Because MFR is an appropriate therapy used for the treatment of fascial densification and soft tissue adaptations, scars and adhesions as a result of injury or surgery can be treated effectively with many of the MFR approaches in this book. (See chapter 10 for scar tissue management techniques.) However, be sure to wait between six to eight weeks before performing MFR over a scar; prior to that time, work can be carried out above and below the incision site.

Cancer

MFR is an appropriate therapy for those with cancer. Over the years there have been conflicting opinions regarding the safety of performing massage on clients with cancer. However, it has been proven that bodywork in general promotes wellness and relaxation in these clients. MFR can be performed on clients who are in remission from cancer and those who are undergoing both chemotherapy and radiotherapy. However, working with people with cancer often requires approval from the client's general practitioner (GP) or oncologist, and it's advisable that therapists check with their own insurers directly.

TIP
- MFR can be performed on clients of any age.
- You may be qualified to treat acute injuries; MFR can be used as part of your therapeutic approach at this stage of the injury.
- A full understanding of responses to MFR is vital when treating an athlete or performer with MFR on the day of an event because the treatment may affect muscle power and proprioception. Discuss this concern with the client.
- MFR can play an important role in a training routine for the athlete and those who are training for a physically active job, because it will maintain and increase flexibility and performance.

Equipment and Room Preparation

MFR requires little preparation. However, the following can help clients feel at ease as soon as they enter the treatment room:

- Clean, warm, quiet and comfortable treatment room and music, if required
- Chair for the client and somewhere safe to place belongings
- Coat hanger or hook on the back of the treatment room door
- Robe or dressing gown to use if the client needs to leave the room to visit the toilet
- Consultation form, body diagrams, case notes, spare paper and a pen or pencil

- Sturdy treatment table, preferably adjustable, with a face hole or face cradle (also called a massage table, plinth, or couch)
- Therapist stool
- Two pillows, bolsters, towels or sheets and a blanket for draping the client
- Therapist treatment tools
- Hand sanitiser and tissues
- Spare hair tie or band
- Water for therapist and client

Many therapists use towels as drapes, but most are not big enough to cover the average body. If you need to drape a client, a sheet is far more practical; use one to cover your treatment table and another to cover the client. Sheets are also easier to wash than towels. A couch roll is another thing that is not practical with MFR. Because clients are sometimes in three or four positions during a session, a couch roll can get in the way and usually gets ripped and ends up on the floor.

Treatment table height is important. Most MFR therapists position their tables at approximately mid-thigh, or slightly above, so they can use their body weight during the treatment and optimise their body mechanics. A treatment table that is too high elevates the shoulders, and one that is too low hurts the back and hyper-extends the wrists. Using inappropriate body mechanics to perform the techniques will eventually lead to burnout and aches and pains.

The average treatment table width is around 27 inches (69 cm); anything wider than that, although comfortable for the client, will require you to stretch farther to perform the techniques. This will eventually result in stiffness and soreness. Conversely, treatment tables that are narrow, like some mobile sport tables and beauty couches, do not allow the client to rest without their arms falling over the sides.

CLIENT TALK

I personally don't think it matters whether the treatment table has a face hole, a hole with a bung or plug cut into one end of the tabletop, or a face cradle that fits into holes at the end of the table with a soft foam headrest. With very tall clients, a face cradle offers extra length to the treatment table, but it can get in the way when you sit at the end. A face hole is quicker and easier to use, and makes the treatment table lighter to carry.

Treatment tables also need to be relatively firm. If the top is too soft, you will be pushing into the foam rather than the client's body when palpating. If your table is too firm, you can place a folded single duvet or quilt on top of it or even a camping or yoga mat, which will also make it feel warmer for the client.

One other important consideration for a treatment table for MFR is whether it has a spring locking system. The average treatment table holds around 350 pounds (159 kg). A spring locking system has cables under it to provide extra support and sturdiness. Some treatment tables have extra legs in the middle, which is fine if the table stays in the treatment room but makes it very heavy if you are a mobile therapist. A treatment table with a back lift so the client can sit up is not necessary; this feature makes the table quite heavy, and the extra nuts and bolts can make it squeakier.

When you perform MFR, you are often supporting your client by kneeling, sitting or leaning into the treatment table. Make sure your treatment table can support the client's weight and yours before you kneel or sit on it.

Lastly, the angle of the legs under the treatment table can make the difference between a sturdy treatment table and one that can move easily and be sturdy at the same time. When the legs are at right angles to the base of the table and you lean into the table or position a client so that their weight is on one side of the table, the table can feel as if it might tip. Tables with legs at slight angles that don't extend farther than the tabletop are less likely to tip when moved.

CLIENT TALK

I am a great believer in setting the scene right from start. We discussed this somewhat in the discussion of the initial assessment in chapter 2. Having the best equipment or the best-decorated treatment room in the country won't make you a better MFR therapist. However, providing relevant and accurate appointment details, including what to expect during treatment and what to wear and bring to the session, as well as a clean, functional and presentable treatment room will promote confidence and trust in you and your treatment.

- If you don't have a hydraulic or electric table, consider a hydraulic stool for yourself and have a small step stool under your treatment table that your clients can use to get on and off the treatment table.
- Buy an adjustable shower stool for working on seated clients so that you can ensure optimal body mechanics for both you and your client.
- A single-bed electric blanket on your treatment table will keep your clients warm.

Correct Body Mechanics

Adopting correct body mechanics at all times is vitally important not only to ensure a long and rewarding career but also to provide the best posture and balance for performing MFR correctly. The techniques part of this book (part III) describes proper body mechanics including how to position your hands, arms and shoulders.

Proper body mechanics include the following:

- Using the correct treatment table height or taking care of your body if you work on the floor
- Wearing adequate and appropriate clothing and footwear

- Keeping your head up and your back straight
- Lunging from your legs as opposed to bending from your hips
- Maintaining a centre of gravity to conserve biomechanical energy and also use it to its full potential
- Bringing the physical and energetic power of each technique from your core whilst maintaining a relaxed body
- Making use of the width of your treatment table and positioning clients so you don't have to stretch to perform the techniques
- Engaging the techniques you are performing with your entire body and mind
- Maintaining soft and sensitive hands and allowing them to 'listen' to what they are doing
- Remembering to breathe

CLIENT TALK

At massage school we were taught the terms *earth hook* and *sky hook* to remember to slightly posteriorly rotate the pelvis as if the sacrum were hooked to the earth and to hold the head up as if there were a hook from the top of the head to the sky. This results in keeping the spine straight and protecting the back so we can perform the massage supporting ourselves from our legs. In this way we can use our body weight and not just the strength of our arms and shoulders. The same applies to the performance of MFR. If your treatment table is at the right height, you can bend your knees slightly, flatten your low back by tucking your pelvis underneath you, hold your head up, drop your shoulders and slightly bend your elbows, all of which offer more power to apply the technique so that it comes through your body, down your arms and into your hands.

Always think about how you can perform a technique with the least effort on your body. When performing certain massage techniques, climbing onto the treatment table provides a better vantage point. This is not the case with MFR. Because of the sustained length of time needed to apply MFR with relaxed and focused hands, maintaining a position of kneeling or standing over the client on the treatment table is not conducive to the approach, nor is it safe, especially when the client begins to move spontaneously as a response to treatment. Because MFR is a slowly applied approach, you must be comfortable performing every technique. If you are not comfortable or your arms and hands (and body) are aching or straining, you will never feel what is happening under your hands.

One other thing to remember when applying MFR is to stand as close to the treatment table as you can, even leaning on it if that's more comfortable. Always perform techniques with your arms and hands close to your body; outstretched arms will only make your back and shoulders ache.

• If the table is too high, you will engage your shoulders too much and hyperextend your wrists during the treatment; if it's too low, your back will start to ache.
   • Listening hands (i.e., soft and sensitive hands) are vitally important. If you feel that you are working too hard, you probably are.

Mental Preparation

MFR therapists mentally and physically create a healing environment by setting the intention to connect with their own unconscious minds, emotions and energy for the benefit of the client and the therapeutic process. Bodywork is energetic. MFR is about releasing restrictions that have been hindering the flow of energy and creating physical, mental and emotional pain and discomfort.

Your intention, as a therapist, is twofold. First, you need to carry the intention to prepare yourself to perform the treatment to the best of your ability; second, you need to actively set an intention to connect with your client physically, emotionally and mentally whilst staying open to any outcome without judgement. Your intention has to be met with appropriate action—that of the application of the technique—otherwise it becomes redundant.

Athletes, competitors and musicians, among others, take time to prepare themselves mentally and physically before they step out in front of a crowd. Therapy should be no different. Although stretching and warming up may be a normal activity for you, make sure also to take the time to check in with yourself to see how you are feeling and whether you are preoccupied with your own clutter. Being preoccupied will affect the therapy you are about to offer your client. In addition to checking in with your mental state, you should also focus on listening with your hands and tuning in to both the physical and mental components of your client.

MFR promotes listening, feeling and following the physical and emotional aspects of any injury. Therefore, you need to be responsive to where the clients are and what they are feeling on that particular day. This allows you to work with them, not on them. You should also encourage the clients to meet you in the process at least halfway by asking them to become aware of or to concentrate on their own body. By doing this you are establishing a therapeutic relationship as well as enhancing the MFR process.

Many people use the terms *grounding* or *focus* for the process of setting, and acting on, the intention to create a space and prepare themselves to treat clients. These terms can also involve the process of mentally and physically connecting with the natural environment as opposed to being directed by the mechanical, and even toxic, arena of today's busy lifestyles. In practice, grounding, focusing and intention involve actively, mentally and consciously focusing on keeping yourself comfortable, receptive and intuitive whilst maintaining an open and responsive connection with your client during the session.

You do not know what will unfold in the treatment session. You have to keep your eyes and ears open and feel with listening hands so you can work with what is given on that day. If you go into a session with an agenda, then you have not listened, looked at or felt what is going on in the human being standing in front of you who is trusting you with their health.

Grounding yourself can be done in a number of ways. Some therapists repeat a mantra; others have plants or candles in the room that they mentally connect with or focus on. Still others have a familiar routine of tuning in to their own bodies by kinaesthetic awareness, and some simply glance at the sky through the window or feel their feet connect with the floor. Find something that allows you to connect with every part of your body so you feel comfortable, soft and receptive before placing your hands on your client.

Set an intention to be receptive and open to what is offered to you without judgement. Logic won't work; if it did, this client would most likely have been 'fixed' by now. Allow your intuition to grow, and follow and feel what is under your hands. This will help you let go of the need to fix anything. Every therapeutic application should be carried out with intention and grounding. It is so important to look after your own body whilst performing any therapy; otherwise, it will be you on the treatment table next.

CLIENT TALK

Do you ever worry that you are not providing enough techniques with the right amount of pressure in the correct amount of time so that clients feel they have received their money's worth? Being scared that clients might think you're not good enough is common among therapists. To help with this, keep in mind that you can only work with what is given. Clients may only be able to offer you a slightly more soft and relaxed body to work with because that is all they are capable of, but if you work well with what is given, you will always create change.

Therapist and Client Communication

Think of a gifted musician whose feeling of connection between body and mind connects with her love of the music, enriching how she plays her instrument. She is completely immersed in how the music makes her feel and where it takes her. Not only that, but she connects with her audience so that receptive listeners can feel her emotion. Her experience is not just about being a musician; it is about being a true artist. In MFR, technique is the bow, and the client's body is the instrument. Your skill in using the bow and how you feel and play the instrument is what differentiates good MFR from great MFR. Just as reading music is different to playing it, learning a technique from a book is different to applying it. Your experience, awareness, skill and intuition grow the more you feel and receive the work, attend workshops and connect with your clients to make every treatment unique.

The art of MFR involves bringing your grounding and intention to what you feel, see and hear from your client. Through your touch and dialoguing skills, you make a therapeutic connection. Encourage your clients to connect with their own bodies and with your hands whilst you sense, feel and follow, without force, what is going on in their bodies so that you work together to facilitate change in the tissues.

This shared state of inner awareness allows both therapist and client to connect to a natural heightened state of consciousness called the hypnagogic state, which occurs between wakefulness and sleep. In this state we are more open, sensitive, receptive and creative, yet incredibly rested. Our irrational boundaries and illogical and outdated belief systems can give way to moments of insight in which solutions can be found. Many therapies and bodywork styles promote this state in varying degrees; to this, the MFR approach adds intention, therapeutic dialoguing and the sensitive application of the techniques, all of which offer great benefits to both therapist and client.

To facilitate this state of communication and connection, try to avoid the following:

- General chitchat regarding the weather, news, TV programmes or sports. Such topics can bring clients back into their analytical, logical left brains, breaking the therapeutic connection.
- Too much therapeutic dialoguing. Talking too much about what is happening in the therapy can have the same effect as general chitchat. Constantly reporting what's moving or releasing, what's stuck or how well the client is doing can become irritating to the client.
- Drawing the client's attention to things happening outside the treatment room. This, too, can interrupt the hypnagogic state.

Bringing your intention, grounding, communication and connection together along with the physical application of techniques provides limitless opportunities for intuition and insight to come to the fore. The more you can engage this process, the more you can learn through the work, the more you can experience and the more your clients will benefit.

Effects of and Responses to MFR

The effects of receiving MFR, and what it feels like during treatment, can be quite varied; this is another reason MFR isn't protocol or recipe oriented. The responses of the client either during or after treatment, or both, can be both physical and emotional, evoke memories from the past or play out a story of a symbolic nature.

Asking the client to describe what they are feeling, to encourage interoception, or noticing during an MFR treatment is quite important. To be able to describe their experience, the client has to concentrate on their body and not on the external environment. This concentration, or feeling into one's own body, is part of the client–therapist connection and builds a sense of self in the client. The client can only describe what they are aware of. If they are not aware of their body, their ability to take part in the client–therapist connection will be limited, and you will have less to work with.

Like most remedial therapies, MFR can elicit what we call therapeutic pain. Some students tell me that they have been trained to stop working as soon as the client reports any pain or discomfort. I believe that it's important to distinguish therapeutic pain from work that is painful to receive and that may cause further damage. MFR will not injure the client, although it can be painful for two reasons. First, MFR is thought to break up cross-linkages between the collagen and elastin fibres, restoring normal resting length. The sensation that normally comes from this process can feel like a burning under the skin. Some clients think this sensation comes from their skin being overstretched, but it is actually from the effect of cellular changes, inflammatory responses and the activation of the sensory nervous system. You need to describe what is happening so your clients understand that nothing is wrong, that the technique is working, so they won't be fearful of what they are feeling. Second, MFR may be perceived as painful when body memory, thoughts and emotions bubble to the surface. Although the client may experience this as pain, it is body memory that an experienced therapist can help guide them through.

If you are performing a technique and the response the client is experiencing becomes painful not because you are doing anything wrong but because of the sharpness of the fascial changes, always guide the client to ask you to lighten up your pressure, because treating the tissue with the client bracing against the discomfort is counterproductive.

Another common occurrence during an MFR treatment is red flare. This is a creeping, stretching, tingling and twitching sensation under the skin or the skin becoming pink (sometimes called hyperaemia or a vasomotor response). This is thought to be as a result of the reorganisation of the collagen and elastin fibres and the viscosity of the ground substance resulting in vasodilation.

Red flare (see figure 3.1) can occur in the area you are treating and also distant to where the therapist's hands are. This is because when one area changes, subsequent areas along the same line of pull or bracing pattern change also. Red flare indicates areas that should be subsequently treated to maximise the results of the therapy.

The following are some normal responses that can occur from a physical or emotional release, or both, during an MFR treatment session:

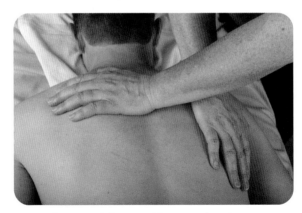

Figure 3.1   Red flare visible on a client's upper back in response to MFR.

- Breathing changes
- Skin colour changes (pallor to flushed)
- Sweating
- Shivering, trembling, vibrating or shaking
- Local or full-body movement often called unwinding
- Emotional release such as laughter, crying, anger, joy or fear

The client may be aware of feelings that occur distant to where your hands are. When this happens, you have the opportunity to re-emphasise the three-dimensional, completely continuous nature of the fascial matrix and the importance of the MFR approach to the client. Explain that as you work and treat one part of the restricted matrix with the heat, weight and pressure from your hands, other restricted areas follow suit and begin to yield under your touch.

CLIENT TALK

Having students at workshops feel this three-dimensional tissue change for the first time is such a rewarding experience. Their eyes light up in an 'aha' moment as they recognise that they are actually facilitating a system-wide change in the client's tissue.

Clients who feel changes in their body for the first time, especially when it is distant to where the therapist's hands are, are more interested and intrigued than anything else. Some clients have felt pain and discomfort for such a long time that feeling something positive is quite a revelation.

Some clients express themselves physically and emotionally during treatment, whereas others start to become emotional but stay very still. Encourage your clients to feel and express what is happening as much as they can because this allows for a change to occur in every aspect of the body. As clients gain a deeper understanding and trust in you and the MFR approach, they will be more willing to express what they are feeling.

The following are some effects that clients may experience after treatment:

- *Therapeutic pain.* This is what we call body stiffness or tenderness post-treatment. It is similar to the stiffness you feel after you have done more than normal physical work.

- *Better sleep.* This is due to less pain and tension.

- *Lethargy.* Clients can feel 'washed out' after treatment. Holding on to huge amounts of tension can be exhausting. As the tension changes, the body is able to show how exhausted it has been from having to hold on.

- *Less painful menstruation cycles.*

- *Old aches and pains.* As layers of restriction and tension change, old injuries that were not adequately treated become uncovered. This process of peeling back the layers reveals both the physical and emotional aspects of all injuries.

- *Energised.* The client feels an increase in energy due to the reduction of tensional loads on the body.

In reality, any experience can be a response to treatment, and responses differ greatly from client to client. I can give you some of the more common responses, but a comprehensive list would be impossible. Remember never to judge your clients; rather, let them know that what they are experiencing is right for, and unique to, them. Any response is a good response, and all should be accepted and respected.

Commonly Asked Questions and Concerns of Therapists

WHAT AM I SUPPOSED TO BE FEELING?   This goes back to the notion of intention. Allow yourself to feel what you are feeling, not what you can't feel. Allow the client's body to meet and respond to your hands; otherwise, you will work too hard.

WHY AM I NOT FOCUSING MY TREATMENT ON THE AREAS OF PAIN?   MFR is a full-body approach. The fascial system, when restricted, pulls and twists, creating pressure and tension that affect pain-sensitive structures throughout the body. Even though the client's shoulder may be in pain, the restriction may be farther down the body, creating a line of tension up into the shoulder. If you stand flexed at the hips with your arm outstretched holding a bucket of water, your arm and back will ache first. No amount of rubbing or strengthening of your back will resolve your pain; all you have to do is release the tension by putting the bucket of water down.

HOW MUCH PRESSURE SHOULD I USE?   It's not how much pressure you use but how much resistance you feel that is important. MFR promotes feeling for and then waiting at the barrier of fascial resistance and not forcing that barrier. Every client is unique, and each one will teach you something new.

HOW LONG SHOULD A SESSION BE, AND HOW OFTEN SHOULD I SEE A CLIENT?   Initial sessions need to be longer than other sessions to give you time to complete the consultation and assessment process. Generally, sessions are from one to two hours in length and are scheduled close together to facilitate breaking habitual holding and bracing patterns of the fascial network.

HOW MANY SESSIONS WILL A CLIENT NEED?   Treatment takes as long as it takes. Every client is unique. If it took 10 years to get this way, the client won't change overnight. However, the client should begin to feel changes as a result of one to three sessions. Some clients reach a plateau in which the body is reorganising and taking its time to get used to the new feelings. Don't get discouraged by this; things will start to move again.

HOW CAN I INTEGRATE MFR INTO MY OTHER TREATMENT MODALITIES?   If you have never performed MFR before, I suggest that you practise two or three techniques from this book on friends, colleagues or suitable clients so you can begin to experience and develop a felt sense of awareness. Further learning and experience can be obtained by attending a workshop or receiving MFR treatments, or both, especially if you are not currently insured to practise remedial therapy. If you already have previous MFR experience, use this book to add insight to your skills, deepen your kinaesthetic touch and expand your knowledge as you develop your own style of MFR.

Closing Remarks

MFR is an experiential therapy. In reality, it cannot be fully learned or taught. It is an intuitive, thought-provoking therapy due to the varying responses clients offer, and it is often regarded as an art form that provides opportunities to work with clients to help them achieve profound positive changes to their physical and emotional well-being.

Each client brings new challenges and learning experiences. Your task is to set an intention to facilitate the process whilst remaining grounded. Avoid judging, leading or analysing; rather, focus on supporting and facilitating the treatment process.

Quick Questions

1. Can MFR be performed on pregnant ladies?
2. What is the difference between local and global contraindications?
3. Should you bend over the treatment table to perform MFR, or should you keep your back straight?
4. Why is communication with the client during the treatment process important?
5. Why is avoiding general chitchat important during the MFR session?

PART II

MFR Applications

This part of the book introduces you to the experience of feeling fascia, which is different to feeling muscle. Chapter 4 offers descriptions of tissue mobility tests that will help you find fascial restrictions. It also describes rebounding, an oscillatory approach that is a great tool for finding and feeling for tissue dysfunction by noticing a lack of fluidity as you gently rock your client's body. Chapter 5 describes the MFR techniques and how to perform them, and offers suggestions for combining techniques for greater effectiveness. It also addresses the use of therapeutic dialoguing to help your clients feel what is happening to their bodies during an MFR treatment session.

Palpatory and Physical Assessments

In the field of Western medicine, the more complicated the test, the greater the amount of scientific research focused on it and the more credible it is. Such tests thus carry far more authority and credibility than any physical palpatory test or simply believing what we feel.

Chaitow recounted the thoughts of Craig Liebenson DC and Karel Lewit MD:

> The skill in which patients are diagnosed and treated in the field of manual medicine requires both science and art. Western medicine has led the way of developing a hands-off, high-tech medicine. (Chaitow 2010)

Despite the credibility given to complex medical tests, becoming familiar with palpation is fundamental to any hands-on therapy. Therapists need to know what is under their hands, not just the basic anatomy but also the character of the tissue and its rhythms and fluid movements. Being able to palpate tissues effectively and to notice levels of tissue tension, thermal abnormalities, inflammation and oedema offers the therapist an opportunity to accurately assess the degree of restriction and apply appropriate treatment.

Palpatory Assessment

A palpatory assessment takes place when you use your palpation skills and begin to apply MFR techniques. This evaluation should be performed on every client in every session. Palpation of the client's body can be performed both with the client in standing position and lying on the treatment table. Because the structure of the body is less affected by gravity when lying on the treatment table, palpation can be more accurate in this position. The position makes it easier to locate any tight, hard, cool and hot areas, which can be signs of restriction.

The following are things to look for in a client evaluation that occurs on the table:

- Tissue equality, bounce and end-feel in all directions (mobility)
- Tissue temperature
- Tissue drag
- Areas that are hard or tender

CLIENT TALK

Some therapists believe that it is important to discuss what they see and feel with the client before treatment commences. I do this whilst applying my first MFR technique, not only because it saves time, but also because I can encourage the client to feel what I am doing. Other therapists wait until the end of the session to discuss their findings, as well as the results from the session. Try it both ways and see what feels right to you. Your clients may prefer one way over the other, so take that into consideration.

The objectives of palpation are to detect the following:

- Abnormal tissue texture (turgescence, elasticity, oedema, clamminess, roughness, dryness)
- Thermal abnormalities (heat and coolness)
- Symmetry versus asymmetry
- Range of tissue mobility

Over the years various ways of palpating have been suggested, including with the sides of the hands, the fingers and the entirety of the hands. Most important, however, is teaching your hands to feel, how to 'think', how to 'see' and then letting them touch. Barnes suggests that you allow your hands to listen to what is going on underneath them so they can tell your mind what they are feeling as opposed to what you logically think they should be feeling.

The process of MFR involves the use of the entirety of the hands for both palpating and performing the techniques. The reasons for this are both to use a larger surface area for gathering information because the hands have a high density of tactile sensory receptive fields and to convey empathy, caring and trust to the client. These feelings are more effectively communicated with the entire hand than with the fingers.

How you touch with your hands is also important. The contact needs to be soft and relaxed yet firm enough so you can feel what is happening under your hands. The touch also needs to be long enough to collect information—not just a brush with the fingertips, but sustained contact.

At this stage, I will discuss only palpation of the client's tissue and some important bony landmarks in standing. You can perform palpatory and postural assessments in many ways. This chapter includes easy assessments that are appropriate for an MFR treatment.

How the tissue looks, feels and moves is something most therapists forget to notice before they start treating. Not only do hypertonicity, tension and temperature provide clues to where restrictions might be, but they also give you something to compare against when you are assessing treatment outcomes.

Mobility refers to the ability of tissues to move and glide. Palpation is the process of using your hands to feel whether a tissue is tight, hard, tender, hot or cold and clammy. You will also feel where the tissue feels stuck to its underlying and surrounding structures and where it has freedom of movement in all directions. This information provides clues to the underlying musculoskeletal and fascial restrictions.

When the body is injured, many processes kick into gear to protect and repair the injured area. In the acute stages of an injury, an increase in circulation makes the tissue feel warm, and an increase in tissue fluid, or oedema, makes the tissue feel boggy or spongy. Tenderness and sensitivity also usually occur in the local area.

A chronic injury can be an acute injury that has not been treated correctly or at all. It can also occur because of a repetitive misuse, overuse or disuse injury, resulting in chronic tissue holding patterns and inflammation. An example is habitual poor posture that results in postural muscles adapting by shortening and contracting and phasic muscles adapting by weakening and lengthening (Page, Frank, and Lardner 2010). When this happens, the fascial network binds down (densification) to support where muscles cannot. The feel of tissue suffering from chronic dysfunction is hard, tight, rough and immobile because of the fibrotic tensional lines of dysfunction below the site. Chronic dysfunction can cause tissue to feel cold, clammy and hypersensitive as a result of ischaemia (deficient supply of blood to carry nutrients and remove toxins) and hypoxia (oxygen deprivation), or to feel hot and tender as a result of inflammation (an increase in blood supply and tissue fluid).

It is important to add here that trauma, both physical and emotional, can also be the cause of chronic pain. In addition to the physical adaptations of soft tissue to a trauma or injury, emotional trauma lives within the tissues and can be detected by the experienced hand. Such tissue often feels as if it is pushing you away, or it may be vibratory to the touch or exhibit other characteristics.

Many therapists are trained to sense the electromagnetic qualities of the tissues using off-the-body scanning to assess for tissue dysfunction of both a physical and emotional nature. Others assess whilst maintaining physical contact at all times. MFR uses a variety of assessment approaches; it is most important that you use the skill that feels right for you.

A feeling of either heat or coolness on your client's skin is a notification that tissue restriction and dysfunction (having already ruled out tissue infection and inflammation in your consultation, which are contraindications) have altered the tissue respiratory and circulatory processes. Before assessing the temperature of your client's skin, it is important that you notice the temperature of your own body compared to that of your client. When palpating for heat and coolness, always use the same hand so that you have a benchmark from which to work. Some therapists suggest using the back of the hand to feel for temperature changes. I don't think it matters as long as you note the difference in temperature between one side of your client's body and the other.

You are also looking and feeling for equality in the tissue, checking whether the tone is the same on both sides of the body. You may notice that one calf seems thicker and tighter than the other, one-foot arch feels flatter than the other, or one shoulder seems more rounded than the other. This occurs when the body is meeting the demand of the tension imposed on it as well as when it is making habitual postural adaptations. Certain areas thicken and shorten in response to stress and repetitive strain, whereas other areas lengthen and strain to maintain balance. The practical applications that follow contain instructions for conducting a general palpation assessment, as well as tips for the direct palpatory assessment of three areas. Ask the client to give you feedback when you perform this assessment, and always note your findings.

Practical Application: General Palpatory

Before you actually place your hands on the client, let's recap how to prepare to use your hands and body as assessment and treatment tools. You need to make sure that you are physically and emotionally comfortable, calm, composed and receptive, without judgement. You also need to convey a sense of competence, trust and nurturing with your hands to continue your established therapeutic relationship from the initial assessments. Review the steps of a visual postural assessment in chapter 2 before undertaking a palpatory assessment.

1. Follow the visual postural assessment by explaining to your client that whilst they are standing you are going to use gentle but firm hands to palpate their body, feeling for equality in the skin and underlying soft tissue. You can start at the client's feet and work up to the head, or vice versa.

2. Perform your assessment from the posterior, anterior and both lateral views.

3. Feel first for temperature. Using the same hand, compare the right side of the body to the left.

4. Take your time as you feel for whether the client has even temperatures. If you notice an inequality, ask the client if they have had any injury or feel any discomfort in that area, and make note of your findings.

5. Now feel for areas of the client's body that feel tight or tender in relationship to the same areas on the opposite side of the body.

6. Gently squeeze the tissue between your thumbs and the palmar side of your fingers.

7. Take your time assessing up and down the client's body, always comparing right to left.

8. Notice if one part of the body feels harder or thicker than the same part on the other side.

9. Take into consideration the client's activity level, occupation and injuries that may have caused compensatory patterns (noting the length of time since any injuries).

10. When you gently palpate by squeezing with your hands, ask the client what that feels like, and make note of the response.

11. If you find a distinct difference in palpation between the right and the left sides (e.g., the upper trapezius muscle at the shoulder),

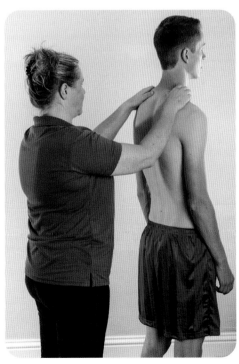

then at some point during treatment you would apply MFR techniques to that area. On retesting after the treatment the client should feel a more equal sensation on both sides.

12. Notice whether anything other than thermal discrepancies or tissue tension draws your attention. Ask the client what they are feeling in that area. You may have found an area of restricted energy or emotion.

13. Take note of your findings.

Practical Application: Foot Palpatory

1. With your client in standing, feel under the medial arch of the feet.
2. What do you feel?
3. Are both arches the same height from the floor?
4. If one arch feels lower to the floor than the other, make a note of this.

A fallen arch can mean many things; it could be the cause of dysfunction higher up the body, or it could be a result of a pelvic imbalance or a leg length discrepancy. Suffice to say that at this stage you can't really know why there may be a fallen arch. Take note of it so that in your post-treatment assessment you can check to see whether it has normalised.

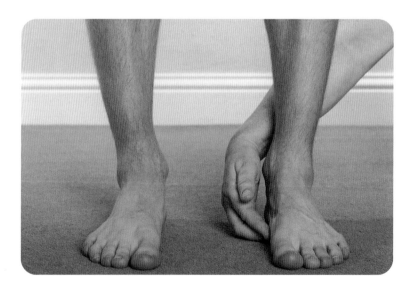

Practical Application: Pelvis Palpatory

Now let's look at four bony landmarks of the pelvis.

1. Palpate for the client's right and left anterior superior iliac spines (ASIS). The ASIS is a prominent bony landmark on the anterior aspect of the pelvis. You can also ask the client to find these bones for you.

2. These bony landmarks should be level right to left.

3. Place your thumbs or fingers on the ASIS and note whether one is higher or lower than the other. To do this, you may need to kneel down in front of the client.

4. Write down what you see.

5. Move around to the side of the client so that you can palpate for the posterior and anterior parts of the pelvis.

6. You are using the ASIS at the front and the posterior superior iliac spine (PSIS) at the back, which are two prominent bony landmarks in the posterior pelvis.

7. To find the PSIS, find the client's dimples at the base of the spine where it articulates with the sacrum.

8. Drop your fingers slightly inferior and lateral to the dimple, where you should find a bony prominence; this is the PSIS.

9. The PSIS and the ASIS on the same side should be equal in height.

10. On women, the ASIS can be slightly lower than the PSIS, but in general, these same-side bony landmarks should be level.

11. Again, make note of your findings.

12. Move around again to kneel behind the client.

13. Palpate to find both dimples at the base of the spine, then drop your fingers slightly inferior and lateral on both sides to find the bilateral PSIS.

14. Finding the PSIS can be quite challenging on some clients. Having the client slowly bend forwards and flex the spine and hips can make finding these bony landmarks slightly easier.

15. Notice whether one PSIS looks higher or lower than its counterpart.

16. Again, make note of your findings.

17. Now perform the same assessment on the client's other side by palpating and noting the difference or similarity in height between the ASIS and PSIS.

You now have four palpatory assessments of the pelvis. The pelvis is thought of as a bowl that has to hold its contents level and equal. When it does, it is called the 'circle of integrity'. When these four points are not equal, dysfunction and imbalance occur, which present in every other part of the body. This body-wide effect occurs not just because the pelvis is in the middle of the body, but also because the entire three-dimensional fascial matrix is completely continuous and maintains its integrity through the pelvis. The bones themselves don't decide to become unbalanced; they are merely spacers in the tensional soft tissue framework. Rather, the soft tissues react to the forces of gravity, poor posture, trauma and inflammation and pull the bones out of alignment. Although you have used the bony landmarks to assess structure, you're also reading the tensile forces that have caused imbalance. The pelvis is capable of rotating to the right and to the left through a vertical axis, tilting anteriorly (the two ASIS move forwards and down) and posteriorly (the two ASIS move backwards and up) through a transverse axis. The pelvis is also capable of tilting to the left (the right side of the pelvis moves superior and side bends to the left; some therapists call this a right upslip) and to the right (the left side of the pelvis moves superior and side bends to the right; some therapists call this a left upslip) through a sagittal axis.

Now feel the tissues above, below and around the pelvis. What areas feel tight and tense, and what areas look thicker or fuller? The anterior thigh often feels tighter and looks thicker on the side where the ASIS is lower than the ASIS on the opposite side. The tightening of the tissue pulls the pelvis forwards and down on that side. Conversely, the PSIS on the same side may be higher relative to the opposite PSIS. As the ASIS is pulled forwards and down, it pulls the same-side PSIS upwards and forwards like a wheel. However, we must bear in mind that any issue is never just about one thing, bone or muscle; the issue is function versus dysfunction in the entire structure.

Because the pelvis is in the middle of the body, balancing it will help balance everything above and below it. There are many excellent MFR techniques for creating balance above, below and through the pelvis. It's always a good idea to work all around the pelvis and then reassess your client in standing. You will often

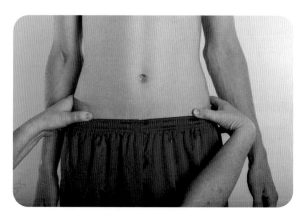

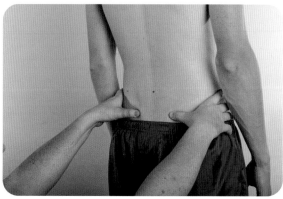

see a great difference in shoulder height and pelvic symmetry, and the client will often report feeling more balanced through the legs and feet. Subsequently, look for the next greatest imbalanced area, treat there and reassess.

At this stage, try not to pass judgement or make logical sense out of what you see and feel. Often what you see in a standing postural assessment is a compensatory pattern and a symptom of the client's dysfunction. This palpatory assessment is simply a way to look and feel for information to help you with the treatment process.

Practical Application: Shoulder Palpatory

The shoulders are often an area of tension and discomfort, and in most clients they are not level from right to left. Dysfunction in this area is often due to overloading of the tissues as well as a compensatory pattern from dysfunction and imbalance lower down in the body.

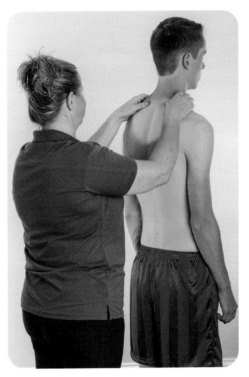

1. Does one shoulder look higher or more forward than the opposite shoulder?

2. Does one shoulder feel tighter than the other?

3. Is the client's head pulled off its central axis towards one shoulder?

4. Does one side of the neck feel tighter to the opposite side?

5. Take note of what you see and feel.

TIP
- Make sure your treatment room is warm, because the client may have to stand for quite a while during your standing postural and palpatory evaluation.
- Notice whether your client can stand still during the assessment. Fidgeting and twitching can be signs of pain as much as changes in skin colour can be a sign that the client is getting cold. Notice whether the client begins to sway in any direction; this can be a sign of system dysfunction and loss of proprioception as the body continually shifts to find balance and stability.
- Everything you see and feel in your palpatory assessment must be compared after treatment. An imbalance is never the result of just one thing in isolation.
- Always be slow and diligent with palpatory assessments; it takes time to feel and listen to another's body.
- After every technique or assessment, remove your hands slowly and gently from the client's skin.

Tissue Mobility and Glide

The assessment for tissue mobility takes place with the client lying on the treatment table. Palpating the body out of gravity provides clues as to where the person is unnecessarily bracing and thus promoting imbalance and dysfunction.

In this assessment you will use your intelligent touch in the same way you did in the standing palpatory assessments, but this time you are feeling for tissue bounce, end-feel and resistance to movement, or in other words, tissue mobility. You will also look at the bony landmarks the way you did in your standing assessments. Any of the thermal or tissue tension tests can be performed in the supine and prone positions in addition to, or instead of, in a standing position.

I have previously mentioned the term *end-feel*, which is applied to anatomical structures at which the available range of motion of a joint or muscle meets resistance. In the context of soft tissue and fascia, the end-feel, or tissue barrier of resistance, is where you feel the give or movement of the tissue stop, which signifies a restriction. We will go through this in more detail when you actually start to perform MFR techniques. For now, you will be leaning into the tissue and noticing the tension, and comparing the right and left sides of the body.

For example, the leg, which felt more tense than its counterpart in your palpatory assessment, would be a good place to apply an MFR technique and then retest for equality. Performing a tissue bounce and end-feel test on the thighs is a good learning experience for this mobility test, but these tests can be performed anywhere on the body. With this test you must take into consideration the give, or resistance, of your treatment table and the area of the body you are performing the test on. It is not easy to perform this test on the shins, but it can be performed on the backs of the legs, gluteal area and hips, back, shoulders, arms, ribcage and abdomen in the same way as on the thighs.

Next you are going to test for tissue glide. Lack of glide signifies a restriction and also offers information as to where the restriction is. The area of restriction can then be treated with an MFR technique to restore freedom of movement. Each layer of continuous tissue from the skin to the core and through to the other side is like a layer of an onion. Each layer is in direct communication with its neighbour through the intricate weaving and supportive fibres of the fascial network. Each layer can glide on its neighbour; however, when a restriction is present, the gliding process is hindered and in some cases the layers become completely glued together where fascia's ground substance has solidified and the collagen and elastin fibres have become stuck together, rather like Velcro (hook and loop tape). As with the tissue mobility assessment, I have chosen an area of the body (the upper back) to experiment on that tends to be easier to work with than other areas are. You can use this technique with both hands to assess the differences and similarities of tissue on the right versus left side of the body, or with one hand to assess tissue restriction in any area of the body. You can be even more specific by using your fingers instead of your whole hand.

Before you apply any touch, remember to ground yourself so that you become soft, receptive and relaxed. Also remember to set the intention of working to the best of your ability without judgement. These topics are covered in the chapter 3 sections Mental Preparation and Therapist and Client Communication.

Practical Application: Tissue Bounce and End-Feel

The test for tissue bounce and end-feel is a general mobility test. You will be feeling for where the tissue stops at the end of its bounce and then begins its recoil phase.

1. Have the client lie face up (supine) on your treatment table.

2. First, look at the position the client is lying in, and take note of it. Some clients have no idea that they are lying crooked on the treatment table and will say that they feel quite straight. In standing, the body tries to organise itself around its centre of gravity whilst keeping the eyes level. When the person is lying down, the postural muscles and the body's righting reflexes relax, permitting dysfunctional patterns to become visible.

3. The thigh is an easy place to start this assessment because it has a broad surface area and good tissue depth.

4. Standing comfortably with your body relaxed, place your hands on the client's thigh with your fingers pointing medially towards the opposite leg. Slowly and gently lean your hands into the thigh, directing your gentle pressure down to the floor, transmitting power through your body to where you feel the client's tissue begin to resist your pressure. This should be completely comfortable for the client and very easy for you to do.

5. Notice whether you can feel a subtle barrier of resistance under your hands and what it feels like.

6. Is the tissue hard or spongy? Does it have a soft end-feel, or do you meet the end-feel quickly with a dead halt?

7. Remember what the tissue feels like so you can compare it to the tissue of the other thigh.

8. Apply a repetitive, gentle bounce into the tissue. The rate is approximately two repetitions per second. Lean your hands in again and gently bounce into the tissue with your body weight for about 5 to 10 seconds. This should be enough time to experience a sense of give, or resistance, in the tissue; however, take more time if you need it.

9. Perform this test on the opposite thigh and compare the results.

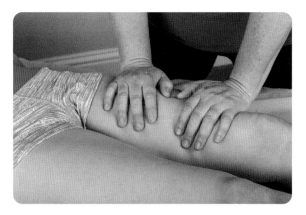

10. Very often, one thigh offers more resistance than the other, which can signify that one leg carries more body weight than the other or is involved in a repetitive strain pattern more than the other is.

Practical Application: Tissue Glide

You can apply this simple technique anywhere on the body. It provides a good indication of general tissue mobility.

1. Have your client lie prone (face down) whilst you stand at the head of the treatment table.
2. Place your hands, skin on skin, onto the client's upper back with one hand on either side of the spine and your fingers pointing down towards the client's feet. You will probably find that your hands are half on the tissue next to the spine and half on the scapulae.
3. Keep your hands soft and allow them to lean into the client's tissue.
4. There should be no discomfort for the client, and you should be able to perform this assessment without using your strength; you should be using just your body weight.
5. Keeping your hands in contact with the client's skin, apply a moderately firm pressure towards the client's feet without slipping on the skin.
6. Notice whether it is easier to push one hand downwards more than it is to push the other.
7. Gently remove your hands and place them back at their starting point.
8. Gently lean into the client's tissue again and drag the tissue, without slipping on the skin, towards the client's head.

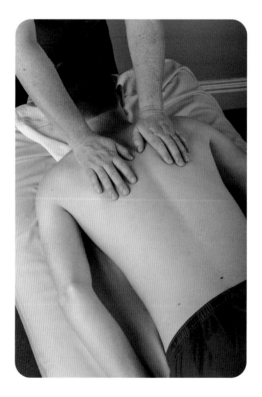

9. Notice whether the drag feels equal.

10. You can perform this test with side-to-side movements as well.

11. When you apply pressure down towards the client's feet and one hand moves farther than the other without slipping, the hand that did not move as far has found a restriction (or more of a restriction than in the tissue on the other side). Because you cannot take the tissue downwards, the restriction is located behind, or superior to, your hand.

12. If you noticed when you dragged the tissue, without slipping on the skin, towards the client's head that one hand travelled farther than the other, the hand that travelled less far has found a restriction (or more of a restriction than in the tissue on the other side). Because you cannot take the tissue downwards, the restriction is located in front of, or inferior to, the hand.

13. You can now apply an MFR technique on the area where you found a fascial restriction and retest the client.

TIP
- Make sure your hands, and your client's skin, are clean and dry before you perform any MFR techniques.
- Most therapists have a dominant side. When performing palpatory assessments, make sure your hands feel equal before performing the drag.
- Take your time practising these assessments. They are essential learning tools and easy and effective diagnostic tools.

Traction and Compression

Traction and compression assessments also use end-feel, but in this case you will be directly assessing the quality of the tissues in and around the client's joints. You will compare the right side of the body to the left side and ultimately evaluate the function and dysfunction of the entire fascial and soft tissue network.

Traction involves gradually and gently lengthening an extremity to its fascial resistance point, or its end-feel. We usually use the arm or leg because they provide a good evaluation not only of themselves but also of the soft tissue throughout the body along the line of pull.

I mentioned previously that fascia is predominantly aligned top to toe in a longitudinal plane. Along these longitudinal planes are horizontal planes that act as supportive slings and dividers of the internal cavities; they also provide functional supports at joints. In tissue glide assessments you traction, or push, the tissue to feel for resistance within the layers below. The same process applies to compressing or tractioning a limb to its end-feel. As you traction the limb, where there is adequate glide and freedom of movement between the soft tissue layers, you should feel, and see, the entire body glide towards you. Where the freedom of the glide stops, or sticks, represents a restriction and an area at which an MFR technique can be applied and a retest performed.

Do you remember the analogy earlier in the book of the tablecloth on the table? Holding the two end corners of the tablecloth and pulling it slowly towards you should generate an even pull through the fabric. If the tablecloth were pinned or nailed to the table, you would not be able to generate an equal and smooth glide of the fabric towards you. In fact, the harder you pull, the tighter the fabric becomes. This is exactly what happens during a traction assessment. As you traction the arm or leg, notice where the movement is fluid, where it becomes less fluid and eventually where the movement ends.

As with the previous two assessments, take the time to make sure your own body is comfortable, relaxed and receptive and that the client is aware of what you're going to do and how you are going to do it. Traction and compression testing involves comparing one side of the body to the other.

Practical Application: Traction

1. With the client supine, stand next to the treatment table facing the client's head and pick up the client's arm so that it is off the treatment table and slightly lateral to their body. Hold the arm gently but securely with one of your hands at the lower arm and the other hand either just below or just above the client's elbow.

2. Apply traction slowly and gently to the arm, tractioning it towards you.

3. Notice the quality of the glide and the tissue end-feel.

4. You should feel a smooth, even glide with a soft, bouncy tissue end-feel.

5. As you gently traction the arm, eventually, the shoulder, neck and head should follow along the line of pull.

6. Encourage the client to relax the head, neck and shoulders so that you can feel the tractioning force through the system without resistance.

7. Release your traction and then reapply the traction to retest the limb.

8. Discuss the sensations with the client and perform the same assessment on the opposite arm, taking note of any discrepancies.

9. Now apply the same test to the client's legs, making sure that the client mentally remains as soft and relaxed as possible.

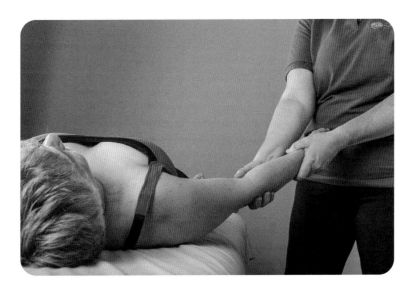

Practical Application: Compression

Compression is the opposite of traction. A compression assessment can be performed with the client supine or prone. It can be done with the right limb followed by the left limb, or vice versa, or by comparing both limbs whilst compressing at the same time. You can assess both legs together whilst standing at the foot of the treatment table, or both arms together by lifting the client's arms up and over the head whilst you stand at the head end of the treatment table.

1. With the client supine, stand next to the treatment table and gently but securely take hold of the client's limb and compress, or push, it up into the joint space, staying sensitive to exploring the tissue to find the end-feel and noticing the quality of the glide through its layers.

2. In some cases, the tissue is so restricted that the compressive force seems minimal and the limb begins to internally or externally rotate.

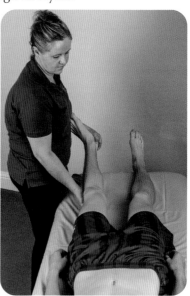

3. When compressing the limb, begin by compressing the most distal joint into the next higher joint, then those two joints into the next higher joint, and so on.

4. The client's body should move with this compressive force. An area of restriction is where the movement ceases and where you begin to lose the connection with that specific area (i.e., where your sensitive hands can't identify the areas you are compressing). Perform MFR techniques at this point and then reassess the limb.

TIP Traction and compression tests are always performed within the client's tolerance. You need to be mindful of the subtle 'felt sense' of the tissues. If the client experiences any discomfort with the traction or compression technique, discontinue the assessment and evaluate the tissues with palpation only.

CLIENT TALK

Students often ask how to increase their kinaesthetic touch and felt sense awareness.

If you practise your palpation skills and some of the fundamental cross-hand release techniques outlined in this book on a few people, you will begin to notice similarities and differences under your hands. Practice is the only way to increase these skills; eventually, it will reap rewards.

Skin Rolling

Skin rolling is not only an effective way to mobilise the tissue but is also a great way to evaluate the skin and the superficial fascia. This assessment and technique mobilise tissue densification and potential adhesions that may have formed between the skin and fascial layers and even internal organs creating a decrease in mobility as well as in circulatory and lymphatic flow.

As an assessment tool, skin rolling is an excellent way of feeling how the skin and superficial fascia are adhered to each other and even to the deeper fascial layers. Skin rolling from the low back up towards the neck may be easier than skin rolling the opposite way. Skin rolling the lateral side of the thoracic area on the left may be easier than on the same area on the right.

You will be working with an area of the body, the upper back, on which it is easy to apply a skin rolling assessment and technique. However, generally, skin rolling can be applied to any area of the body where there is enough tissue to grasp hold of without pinching the skin.

Skin rolling can create a huge circulation rush to superficial tissues, turning the skin a pinker or darker and flushed tone quite rapidly dependant on the skin type. As you lift the skin, you are lifting it away from the underlying tissues where restrictions may be present. Areas that stay a pinker, darker, or a flushed tone often signify where circulation is impeded as a result of a restriction and where you can apply an MFR technique. You can also continue to skin roll around the local area to normalise function. Because skin rolling can be quite tender to receive, it must be done within the client's tolerance level. It is not just about how much tissue you are able to skin roll, but also about the direction and speed of your rolling.

Practical Application: Skin Rolling

Tissue that is not easily rolled between your fingers and thumbs, is tender or turns a pinker, darker, or a flushed tone more quickly than other tissue in surrounding areas signifies a restriction that can be subsequently treated. The client should then be retested.

1. With the client lying prone (face down) on the table, and having told them what you are going to do, stand next to the treatment facing their head. Take a moment to set your intention and ground yourself before placing your hands on the client's body.

2. Begin by gently, but securely, grasping the tissue of the client's back between your finger pads and the thumbs of both hands.

3. You can place one hand on either side of the spine or both hands on the same side of the spine.

4. Roll the tissue over your finger pads with your thumbs, one hand at a time, walking your thumbs forwards and up your client's back to engage more tissue.

5. Notice where the tissue feels stuck or is tender for the client.

6. Repeat the assessment by skin rolling down the client's back by standing closer to the client's head and facing towards their feet.

7. You can also perform the skin rolling assessment across the client's back.

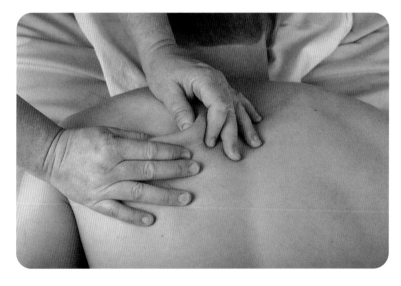

TIP It is easiest to perform skin rolling on the parts of the body where the skin is loose, particularly when you are just learning the technique. There is a bit of a knack to skin rolling. Done wrong, it can feel as though the skin is being pinched. Take your time. The slower you go, the easier it will be to learn the finger and thumb movements and the easier it will be for the client to receive.

Rebounding

Rebounding is a component of the John F. Barnes myofascial approach and is another excellent way to treat and assess the tissues of the body. This section describes the basics of rebounding in relationship to diagnostic testing only, so that you can integrate it into your assessment approach.

Myofascial rebounding uses the feel and rhythm of the body and ultimately the fascial system as an indicator of fluidity and restriction. In our assessment process so far, we have tested for tissue mobility with direct tissue palpation and tissue bounce and drag and by using the limbs as handles to assess how easily the tissues can glide past each other in longitudinal planes. Now we are going to add to these assessments the ease of the tissues, and body parts, to respond to a rhythmic rocking motion applied gently by the therapist's hands.

Practical Application: Leg Rebounding

The arms and legs can be assessed by directly rebounding them. Directly rebounding the torso will not only show fluidity of the torso but will also show the movements and fluidity of the arms and legs as they follow the movement generated from the torso.

1. With the client supine, take the time to establish your intention and ensure that your own body is relaxed and soft.

2. Standing at the client's legs, place both of your flat hands on the client's leg, one below the knee and one above the knee.

3. Lean gently into the tissue and roll the leg in a small movement away from you (medially, or internally) looking for the end-feel of that medial roll.

4. As soon as you notice the end-feel, maintain your contact with the skin but allow the tissue and limb to roll back towards you. As soon as it comes back to its end range laterally, once again roll it medially to its end-feel and continue to rock the limb medially and laterally.

5. The rhythm is about one to two repetitions per second, but this is client dependant. The rhythm has nothing to do with the size of the client; rather, it depends on the bracing and holding patterns in the client's body.

6. As you rock the client's body, notice what else moves and what does not move, especially when you ask the client to become soft and flow with the movement.

7. Wherever the movement does not flow into is a restriction, which can be treated with an MFR technique.

8. Continue to rock the client for about 10 to 20 seconds, and then perform the test on the opposite leg, noticing any differences and similarities.

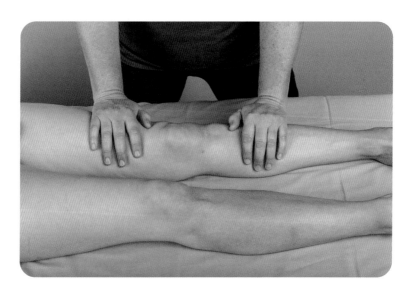

Practical Application: Torso Rebounding

1. With the client supine, stand at the client's hips.
2. Place one of your flat hands on the client's hips and upper leg area at the side closest to you and the other on the client's lateral ribcage.
3. Gently push the client's body away from you until you feel the end of range of the fluid movement. Then, without removing your hands, release your pressure and allow the body to come back towards you.
4. As soon as the client's body finds its fluid end range towards you, push it away from you again, repeating the motion and searching for the rhythm of the client's body.
5. Continue to rock, noticing what moves and what doesn't move.
6. Perform the same assessment by standing on the opposite side of the client's body and notice if there are any differences to the first side.
7. Wherever there is absence of movement is where you should perform MFR techniques and retest.
8. Discuss what you feel with the client, and add your findings to your assessment notes.

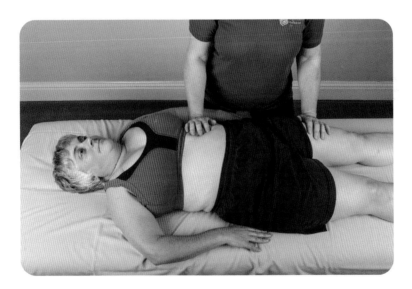

TIP
- Start slowly and feel for your client's rhythm; every client's rhythm is unique. Restrictions, fluidity and energetic flow are different from person to person.
- Rebounding can be performed at any time during the initial assessment or treatment process.
- Rebounding can be performed prone or supine.

Closing Remarks

Although assessments are usually performed at the beginning of a treatment session, there is no harm to integrating them into the MFR session. Take time to perform assessments and evaluations because they not only provide a benchmark of progress but also let the client see and feel how they are benefitting from the treatment.

Quick Questions

1. What does the term *mobility* mean?
2. What does the term *end-feel* mean?
3. What is the full name for the ASIS?
4. What oscillatory assessment approach is used in the John F. Barnes approach to MFR?
5. Can you use palpation in both standing and lying positions?

MFR Technique Approaches

This book describes many different MFR techniques. However, the application of each technique is similar in that each focuses on the client's body resistance, not the pressure that the therapist thinks needs to be put into the tissue. Students often ask how much pressure they should apply. As mentioned before, one of the important aspects of becoming a skilled MFR therapist is to feel the resistance from the client's tissue and apply a pressure that does not force, overwhelm or beat up the tissue. The phrase 'no pain, no gain' has no place in manual therapy because of the increasing amount of evidence of the fascial network's responsibility and role in pain and dysfunction.

When performing MFR, the hands do not slip or glide over the skin. The client's skin must be dry with no oil or lotion, and all techniques must be performed skin on skin, not through drapes, towels or clothing unless necessary for the client's modesty. All the techniques must be applied at the barrier of tissue resistance (end-feel) and held at that barrier for at least three to five minutes to give the client the opportunity to feel and comprehend the responses in their own body and to respond to the treatment, both physically and emotionally. This also gives the tissue time to reorganise and respond in terms of fluid dynamics and mechanoreceptor response.

How to Apply Every MFR Technique

Always prepare yourself, both mentally and physically, to treat a client. You do this by setting, and acting on, a therapeutic goal and using constructive communication and good dialoguing skills. Focus on your sense of touch whilst maintaining a non-judgemental and open-minded approach so that the treatment is client focused. See chapter 3 for a more in-depth discussion of mental preparation and therapist and client communication.

Before you place your hands on a client, be aware of your own body. Make sure you feel comfortable and relaxed in the space you are in and that you have left all of your mental clutter at the treatment room door. You need to bring all of your focus into the treatment room and to be fully present with your intention. Some therapists call this grounding or focusing.

Preparing to Treat Your Client

Before the treatment session, you need to set a clear intention of what you are about to do. That is, you need to approach and work with your client in an open-minded way so you can respond to the needs of the client rather than myopically follow a symptomatic recipe-orientated approach.

Always approach your client's body with interest, empathy, caring and curiosity about what you are going to find. Cultivate an attitude of 'How can I help?' and 'Tell me what you want me to do' in your hands. Every technique is applied slowly and gently from beginning to end, never rushed, never forced. Always feel and search for the tissue barrier and wait for it to soften rather than overwhelm it.

Making a connection with your client is crucial. Having performed the initial intake and gathered personal details followed by the postural and palpatory assessment, explain to the client the technique you are going to apply and where you are going to apply it.

Ask the client to assist in the process by bringing awareness to where your hands are and communicating with their body, in whatever way works for them, to allow their body to soften to your touch. This is because the sense of self, or inner awareness, is the process of interoception of which the fascial system plays a crucial role. This can be as simple as asking the client to allow the body to become soft underneath and around your hands.

All MFR techniques, although applied similarly, involve following and feeling for the unique three-dimensional restrictions in each client's body, making every session completely different to the next. Despite the fact that we have the same musculoskeletal arrangement, we are unique human beings with a unique history, personality and beliefs. Therefore, the way we function is unique to us. This means that we all harbour our own individual framework in the fascial net to support who and what we are. The MFR therapist works with the unique individual client, looking and feeling for the client's own personal lines of dysfunction and function and offering a bespoke treatment to help the client return to a pain-free, active lifestyle.

Tissue Barrier of Resistance

MFR techniques are applied slowly and diligently as you soften into and through the superficial fascia to meet the more resilient, deeper fascia where the restrictions lie. Each technique is applied with intention and without forcing the barrier.

I mentioned in previous chapters the terms *end-feel* and *tissue barrier of resistance*. These terms describe the subtle tissue resistance of the muscular and elastocollagenous component of the fascial web unique to every person. In earlier chapters I mentioned that applying MFR is not about how much pressure you use;

it's about how much resistance you feel. Every technique is applied with 'listening hands'. You apply appropriate pressure for the correct amount of time and follow the tissue as it changes.

The time element is vital to allow the much slower reorganisation of the collagen and the movement of the bound water. From a fascial point of view, the point at which the tissue changes from a relaxed, or soft, state of give to a subtle but definitive state of resistance is called the tissue barrier of resistance. This barrier is where your hands meet the muscular and elastocollagenous barrier of resistance, which must not be forced.

Depending on the technique, the tissue barrier of resistance can be felt in every plane as well as in the direction of the unique pull of restriction through a client's body. We also use the term *depth barrier* to describe the tissue barrier of resistance you feel when leaning into the client's body. As you feel the musculoelastic tissue depth barrier soften, you need to maintain your pressure and take up the slack to meet the next subtle barrier of tissue resistance. In other words, when you feel the resistive barrier melt, apply a little bit more pressure in the direction of the specific technique until you perceive another level or layer of tissue resistance. These barriers can be very subtle. This is the skill of MFR: feeling for and meeting as opposed to forcing the barriers.

Fascial and muscle layers must glide over each other. Imagine you have six slices of bread with butter in between each slice. Your role as an MFR therapist is to lean slowly into the top slice of bread with a small amount of pressure that still allows a degree of glide in the slices of bread below. The MFR techniques should encourage tissue glide. If you push too quickly and too hard, you will pin the six slices of bread together and no glide can occur. As fascia responds to stressors, it will naturally bind down against the pressure applied. This is why all MFR techniques are performed slowly and diligently to avoid the counterpressure of the fascial system. This process of leaning into the tissue is a continuous, subtle pressure for approximately three to five minutes, sometimes longer, to allow both the musculoelastic and collagenous aspects of the tissue to yield and soften.

When you place your hands on the client's skin, lean into the client's body slowly and feel your hands, a loose fist or your elbow sinking into the tissue as if sinking into soft clay or a memory foam pillow. Where this yielding sensation stops and you meet tissue resistance is the depth barrier of tissue resistance or end-feel. As you sit on this barrier, without force, your sustained pressure allows the tissue to respond by softening and yielding. Now lean into the next depth barrier of tissue resistance and wait for it to yield. Follow this process again and again. Because fascia is a three-dimensional matrix, the barrier of resistance can also be felt on multiple planes, all of which you will follow. Because you want to get as deep into the tissue as possible, you should always maintain your focus on the depth barrier of tissue resistance but be aware of fascial resistance and yielding in all directions.

The following is a breakdown of all MFR techniques in simple stages:

- Always perform MFR skin on skin without any oil, wax or lotion.
- Set an intention to make a therapeutic connection with, or to ground, yourself and your client.

- Place your hands gently on the client's body, leaning into the depth barrier of tissue resistance or tractions to meet the tissue barrier of resistance, and wait for a sensation of yielding whilst dialoguing as appropriate with the client.

- Never force the tissue or slip over the skin at any time.

- Gently take up the slack as the tissue softens to the next barrier of tissue resistance.

- Wait at this new barrier for further yielding and softening before taking up the slack to the next barrier. This means that you wait and soften into barrier after barrier.

- Dialogue with the client during the technique, looking for feedback or any responses to and effects of the technique.

- Take up the slack at the point at which every barrier of tissue resistance yields and softens, and follow to the next barrier.

- Disengage slowly from the tissue after approximately five minutes or more, depending on the client.

- Dialogue further with the client for feedback or any other responses to and effects of the technique, which can indicate subsequent areas for treatment.

- Look over the client's body for red flare of the skin (erythema), which occurs with tissue change. This can also indicate subsequent areas of treatment.

Effectively, MFR is a three-dimensional technique that is applied to treat the three-dimensional restrictions within the three-dimensional fascial continuum. As you become more proficient with the techniques, you will find that your hands will begin to follow and become much more fluid with the tissue as it softens as opposed to mechanically applying pressure in various directions.

 • Get comfortable, either standing or seated, before you start a technique.
- Recognise that some clients connect with their own bodies more easily than others do; advise your clients that practice makes perfect.
- Many clients who have experienced long-term chronic pain have disengaged from their bodies to escape the pain. They may need some time to re-engage with themselves physically.
- Do not lead, force or judge; rather, facilitate, follow and support.
- Maintain listening hands at all times. If you feel you are working too hard, then you probably are.
- The superficial fascia feels quite bouncy and soft compared to the denser and firmer deep fascia. Learn to feel and take your intuition past the skin and superficial fascia to engage the subtle nuances of the restrictions hidden in the deep fascia.

TIP • Every technique described in this book can be used as part of all MFR treatments regardless of the client's areas of pain and discomfort. As a result of new research on fascial anatomy, many now accept that pain and discomfort can be caused by fascial restrictions distant to the site of pain.
- MFR has always promoted the concept of finding the pain and looking elsewhere for the cause. Therefore, any technique or combination of techniques can restore

pain-free function. The art of MFR lies not in choosing the techniques to apply to 'fix' the pain but in the kinaesthetic awareness of where restrictions exist coupled with the ability to follow and feel changes in the fluid-filled fascial network.

• Every MFR technique affects the entire three-dimensional fascial matrix; it must be treated as a whole to eliminate the client's pain and dysfunction.

Therapeutic Dialoguing

Dialoguing during MFR treatment is an effective and intuitive tool. It helps the client focus and grow their interoceptive awareness during the treatment and on their body's responses whilst providing valuable feedback for the therapist. Here I describe the simplest and easiest dialoguing methods to facilitate the MFR approach.

MFR is greatly enhanced when both you and your client focus together on kinaesthetic touch. When the client focuses on their own body, they often experience sensations they had not previously been aware of. People who experience pain try to dissociate emotionally from where they feel their pain. In doing so, they also dissociate from the general sensation of their body. If you use words and phrases that make the client think about what they feel, they also have to think how to describe what they are feeling. Often, clients have unconscious beliefs and habitual patterns they have established to protect themselves from pain. Even when the tissues have healed from an injury or they no longer need to use their body in a specific way as a compensation, these unconscious holding patterns have become a habit. Asking the client to focus on their body during treatment is a good way to help the client feel how their body can change so that they realise when they are tightening their body or repeating an unnecessary pattern.

Make time throughout the treatment to ask the client to describe what they feel. Try to stay away from analytical questions that include the words *what*, *when* and *why*, because these encourage the client to analyse and judge their feelings and experiences.

Initially, you might ask the client to close their eyes, which enhances interoception, and to focus on the part of the body where your hands are, allowing it to become soft and relaxed. Use simple words and concepts so the client doesn't have to struggle to understand what they are being asked to do. During the consultation process, pay attention to the way the client describes symptoms. This can provide clues about the client's learning style and whether they are a right-brain person (creative and descriptive) or a left-brain person (logical and analytical, or even visual, auditory, verbal or kinaesthetic). This is a very general description of the characteristics of the right and left brain; however, it can help you formulate your dialoguing to suit the client.

Encourage the client to maintain an awareness and softness in the body as the technique progresses and to notice whether effects occur anywhere else in the body (and to let you know what and where). Responses felt in areas distant to where your hands are placed are areas that require subsequent treatment because they are connected to an injury or body compensatory pattern.

Cross-Hand Releases

Cross-hand release techniques are by far the most important, fundamental and commonly used techniques in the sustained MFR approach. They flow and bind other techniques together and are the best way to learn what the fascial system feels like, which will help you perform MFR more effectively.

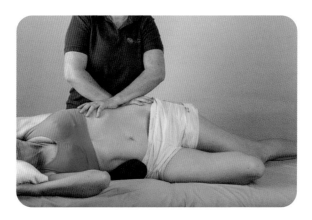

The name of this technique derives from the fact that you cross your hands, usually at the lower arm or wrist, so that your fingers point in opposite directions. Once you have an understanding of how to apply MFR and have learned the application of a cross-hand release technique, you can experiment with hand, and even finger, positioning to obtain the desired tissue changes anywhere on the client's body.

Crossed hands are applied to the client's skin with a gentle, sustained pressure to the tissue depth barrier; feel for tissue resistance in the soft, bouncy superficial fascia. Whilst your hands are applying light pressure, you should be mentally connecting with all of the tissue under and around your hands (and ultimately the entire fascial matrix). The weight of your hands creates a yielding sensation in the skin and superficial fascial layers, as though your hands were sinking into soft clay.

Once you have found the tissue depth barrier, wait at the barrier until it softens and yields so you can apply further gentle, sustained pressure inwards to the next depth barrier of tissue resistance, without force. There is a definitive change to the tissue texture and end-feel of the deep fascia, which can be felt as the superficial fascia yields. The tissue resistance of the deep fascia feels like toffee or chewing gum, as opposed to the butter-melting sensation of the superficial fascia. The deep fascia feels tough, compact and inelastic, providing you with a real sense of being able to lengthen the tissue as it yields to your touch.

As the tissue continues to soften into the deeper layers, you will also begin to feel the tissue yield between your hands. Whilst maintaining pressure at the depth barrier and leaning into the client, separate your hands, or take up the slack between your hands to the end-feel of that dimension as well, without force or slipping or gliding over the skin, thus holding two dimensions of pressure. Now wait for a separation, or lengthening, of the tissue between your hands and facilitate the technique further by once again taking up the slack between your hands to the next tissue barrier. Tissue changes can occur in either an inwards or lengthening direction, or both, which you can facilitate by holding the tissue at the barrier or end-feel, without slipping or gliding over the skin, so that multiple restrictions can change.

Movement can also occur in a third dimension. Whilst maintaining your inward pressure and lengthening between your hands at tissue resistance, you may feel the tissue begin to soften in either a lateral or medial direction or in a twisting motion. Follow with your hands and wait at that barrier, thus stacking three planes, or directions, of movement on top of each other to facilitate a three-dimensional tissue change.

The time needed to perform an average cross-hand release technique is approximately three to five minutes, sometimes more. Because collagen begins to change only at approximately the 90- to 120-second mark, 90 seconds is required to facilitate a lengthening of both the musculoelastic and elastocollagenous fibres. The longer you apply the technique, the more it will affect the entire three-dimensional fascial matrix.

Every cross-hand release is unique. Although the technique itself is applied in a three- dimensional manner each time, the technique follows the untwisting, lengthening and separating of the particular restriction that you follow with subtle, searching hands. Also, the sensations and responses that you and your client experience will feel completely different. Therefore, take time to allow your hands to sink into the client's tissue initially without force and then follow the yielding of the tissue in whichever direction the client offers.

By far the most important aspect of a cross-hand release technique is sensitivity, subtlety and diligence at feeling for tissue resistance. Once you become experienced at the technique, you will learn to feel, follow and listen with your hands, following the directions of tissue change moving through barrier after barrier with the fluid ebb and flow of the system. This encourages the client to relax and soften and to actively participate in the technique. This supports your connection with the client, which in turn heightens the effects of and responses to the technique.

TIP Practising the cross-hand technique will allow you to feel the subtlety of the fascial matrix. You will learn to feel past dense muscular tissue and become aware of the unity of the entire system. This will help you follow the direction offered as the tissue changes as well as begin to feel where restrictions go to and come from.

- Always work skin on skin without oil, cream or lotion, and never force the tissue barrier or slip over the skin.
- Engage and act on your intention, communicate with your client, apply the technique, dialogue as appropriate and wait and follow the tissue response.
- Effective client positioning enhances every technique. No one is ever injured lying flat on a treatment table. Clients need to be treated in various positions in three-dimensional space (prone, supine, side lying, semi-prone, seated and standing) to access the three-dimensional fascial restrictions.
- It doesn't matter whether you cross your right hand over your left or vice versa; however, it is best to alternate to avoid repetitive strain.
- Above all, wait and be patient, and don't try too hard.

Longitudinal Plane Releases

Because fascia is predominantly aligned top to toe, longitudinal plane techniques are used to treat not only the limb being pulled, but they are also used as a lever to access the rest of the body along the vector or line of pull. The easiest way to access longitudinal planes is to use the arms and legs as levers. Arm and leg pulls can be used for both assessment and technique

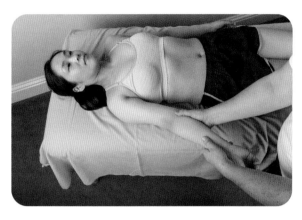

application. The concept of the technique is similar to that of cross-hand releases: take the tissue to the barrier of tissue resistance, or end-feel, without force in three directions of movement, wait at the barrier and follow any tissue changes offered.

To treat joints, their associated soft tissues and the tissues along the longitudinal fascial planes, you will use the barriers present in traction, external rotation and abduction. This is done by lifting the extremity off the treatment table and gently tractioning, or pulling, it to tissue resistance, feeling for the subtlety of the fascial barrier and not the muscular barrier. You will need to lean back slightly to meet the tissue resistance, or end-feel rather than use your strength to perform the technique. This technique then becomes a balancing of your body against the client's, a bit like a children's seesaw. You have to maintain a balance where you are not overpulling but pulling enough so that you can lean back and balance on the resistance of the client's limb.

Maintaining pressure at the tissue barrier, and without slipping on the skin or forcing the barrier, gently abduct the limb to tissue resistance of that movement at the same time. Maintaining pressure at the two previous barriers, add external rotation to the tissue barrier at the shoulder or hip joint. In this way, you are stacking the extremity in three directions of movement.

At this point you need to wait for a yielding and softening of the tissues barrier in any direction and take up the available slack to the next barrier of tissue resistance. Continue to wait, sense and feel until a significant yielding has occurred in all directions.

Most MFR techniques require three to five minutes or more for a lasting result, although arm and leg pulls often take longer because of their anatomical structure. Longitudinal plane techniques performed with diligence and listening hands provide good results not only in the limb but also through the entire body.

You can create tissue change in practically all planes of movement of the hip and shoulder joint by performing arm and leg pulls in supine, prone or side-lying positions. Initially, traction, abduction and external rotation will take the limb out to the side of the client, then into hip and shoulder flexion, followed by adduction and internal rotation as you facilitate tissue change at the joint as the limb crosses over the client's body, creating joint circumduction. When performing the leg pull, to further facilitate the technique, you can maintain the ankle in dorsiflexion through all planes of movement and the subsequent tissue change.

In addition to being excellent techniques for addressing restricted joints, arm and leg pulls also play an important role in creating change in the entire fascial matrix because fascia is predominantly aligned top to toe (longitudinally). By positioning the arm or leg at a certain angle away from the body, you can facilitate change from the point of restriction through the body three-dimensionally to engage any fascial strain pattern that may exist along the line of traction.

As discussed in chapter 4 in the section Traction and Compression, using the longitudinal planes offers an excellent diagnostic approach in the evaluation of tissue and joint restrictions. They are an excellent method of assessing right to left limb similarities and differences as well as feeling with subtle hands where restrictions are present either in the limb or within its line of pull. Such restrictions suggest areas requiring an MFR treatment such as a cross-hand release. This should be followed by a reassessment of the limb.

As in the cross-hand release technique, once you become more experienced at performing arm and leg pulls, you will begin to notice that there is hardly any differentiation among traction, abduction and external rotation. Instead, you will be able to locate the tissue resistance easily and intuit where you need to wait for the fascia to reorganise and the limb to glide to the next barrier of resistance in any plane of movement.

Although working with longitudinal planes involves stacking three planes of movement, these directional planes may be stacked in any order (i.e., not necessarily traction followed by abduction followed by external rotation). In some cases, when you use the traction component, you may be able to discern or intuit that the limb is so tight that compression followed by internal rotation would provide a greater and more beneficial technique for the client than traction followed by external rotation. Developing this ability to discern by feel takes time and experience, but with practice it will happen, and the process will feel effortless. This will be addressed in greater detail in chapter 8, Compression Releases.

In addition to arm and leg pulls, longitudinal plane releases include cervical traction and localised work on the fingers and toes.

 • Take care not to hold the wrist or ankle too tightly; ensure that the client is comfortable with your hold.
- Always wait at the tissue barrier, or end-feel.
- Don't slip on the skin or force the barrier.
- Be subtle and gentle; if you are not feeling anything change, give the limb some slack, because you may be working too hard. With MFR, less is often more.
- Some clients' legs can feel very heavy. Take care to position yourself to support the weight of the leg.
- When performing a leg pull, ask the client to tell you if the knee becomes uncomfortable, because it will be in slight extension. For clients with knee issues or whose knees become uncomfortable, you can perform leg pulls prone or supine, keeping the leg on the treatment table but still employing traction, external rotation and abduction to resistance.

Compression Releases

Because the fascial system is a network of three-dimensional fibres, tissue change can be obtained by lengthening the tissue in multiple directions as in pushing or gliding it away from you or pulling towards you. In effect, compression release techniques are a method of holding the tissue at its tissue barrier, waiting for the tissue change to occur, then taking up the

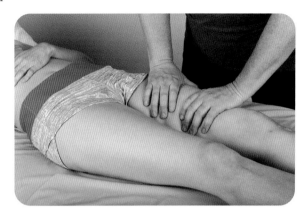

available slack in the tissue and leaning in or pushing or gliding the tissue to the next tissue barrier. In most traditional therapies, we traction or lengthen tissue away from its restriction, which is also the case for many MFR approaches. However, sometimes the tissue is so tight and restricted that tractioning the tissue can feel painful for the client. Compression of the structure will still, in effect, lengthen tissue, because the tissue will still yield to your touch in the same way it does with a traction technique. But more importantly, compression release techniques will help to eradicate habitual, unconscious, physical and emotional holding and bracing patterns. Compression techniques are basically opposite to cross-hand and longitudinal plane releases.

When performing a longitudinal plane release for the arm, traction the tissue to the tissue barrier, or end-feel, and then apply external rotation followed by abduction to the end-feel. With compression techniques, you apply compression to the resistance of the tissues and wait without forcing the barrier or slipping on the skin. Sometimes this is all you need to do for the system to begin to change. Other options are to apply compression to the arm followed by external rotation and abduction to obtain a significant tissue change.

To perform compression of the tissue on the anterior thigh, instead of crossing your hands, place them side by side. Allow them to sink inwards into the client's body to the tissue depth barrier. Then, draw your hands closer together by taking up the slack and following any change offered. Always remember never to force the barrier or slip on the skin.

Compression techniques often yield results in situations in which traction techniques fail. This is not because the preceding techniques were not performed well enough; it's simply that the tissue has a physical and emotional holding pattern that can be better addressed by compression. As with cross-hand release techniques, compression release techniques require on average five minutes, sometimes more, to obtain effective tissue changes.

TIP   When a longitudinal plane or cross-hand release fails to offer results, try a gentle compressive force and then reapply your initial technique.

Transverse Plane Releases

The majority of the fascial planes of the human body are arranged vertically rather than horizontally. A gliding motion is less apparent in the transverse than in the longitudinal plane. Anatomically, certain structural divisions, when tight, act as areas of functional resistance to the natural longitudinal glide of the body's fascial sheets.

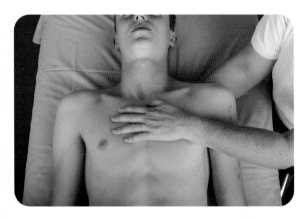

Transverse planes are located wherever there is a predominance of functional connective tissue. The most important transverse fascial planes are found at the pelvic diaphragm, respiratory diaphragm, thoracic inlet and cranial base. These planes also correspond to the levels of spinal transition, which are the greatest areas of stress along the spinal column. Transverse planes also occur at each joint.

To perform a transverse plane release, place one hand, skin on skin, underneath the client, who is lying supine. Then place the other hand directly above your lower hand, again skin on skin. Allow your lower hand to remain soft and supportive whilst the upper hand gently sinks into the client's body without forcing the barrier or slipping over the skin. (This is similar to sinking into the depth barrier in the cross-hand technique.) Invoke your awareness, or concentrate on your soft hands as they contact the client's skin, and wait for a yielding sensation from their tissues that allows you to sink your hands farther into the next barrier of tissue resistance. As the tissue yields and softens, follow and take up the slack in any direction offered. This technique takes approximately three to five minutes, sometimes more. Transverse plane release techniques can be done with the client seated, standing or lying on the treatment table.

Whereas the cross-hand and longitudinal plane release techniques lengthen the tissue, the transverse plane technique compresses the tissue. Because fascia is three-dimensional, it can reorganise in any direction and can move and yield in any direction because it is a single connected network.

TIP Even though transverse plane releases are techniques in their own right, I often describe them akin to a cross-hand release technique through the body. This is because you still have an inward yielding of the tissue from the top hand and a softening of the body down onto your lower hand followed by a side-to-side movement, twisting, spiralling or top-to-toe movement depending on the restriction with which you are working.

TIP Transverse plane release techniques are great techniques with which to commence or end a treatment session. They are a good introduction to MFR and provide good felt sense awareness throughout the body.

Scar Tissue and Adhesion Management

A scar, the result of an injury or surgery, is where the tissue has either healed itself or was repaired by sutures, staples and even dermal glue. An adhesion is the gluing or bonding of sub-dermal tissue to a non-anatomical site as a result of an injury or surgery (Bove et al. 2017).

Because MFR is used as a treatment for injuries, dysfunction and pain, treating scars and adhesions is no different and doesn't require a completely new repertoire of techniques.

The most important thing to consider about a scar is that tissue is repairing, so a six-week wait after the injury or surgery is usually recommended before any techniques can be performed directly on the scar. However, MFR can be performed in other body areas whilst the scar site heals.

The three previous techniques mentioned—the cross-hand release, longitudinal pulls and transverse plane techniques—are all appropriate for scar tissue and adhesions. Cross-hand release techniques can be done over the scar in both a longitudinal and transverse manner, and transverse plane release techniques can also be performed right over the scar site after six weeks.

Scar tissue and adhesion management can also be addressed by skin rolling around the scar, towards it and away from it in all directions. Within the client's comfort level, you can also skin roll the scar, particularly a burn scar. Skin rolling is where you grasp the skin and gently roll it between your fingers and thumbs in a continuous manner. It is an extremely beneficial technique that encourages pliability and glide between the skin and superficial fascia as well as increasing blood flow. Skin rolling, especially over the descending, transverse and ascending colon, is particularly good for clients who have had abdominal surgery.

Two other effective scar tissue and adhesion management techniques involve lifting the tissue, assessing scar tissue glide and taking the tissue to its position of ease, stacking positions of ease on top of each other and then waiting for the tissue to soften. You can also slowly and gently sink into the site of scarring or area of tension surrounding the scar after assessing it for the most tender area. Once you have waited for the tissue tension to subside and the discomfort level to decrease, you then repeat the process in the next most tender area of the scar until you have completed the entire scar.

Myofascial Mobilisations

As mentioned in chapter 1, myofascial mobilisations use a variety of approaches and are typically used to treat muscles and their associated fascial connections.

One method is to apply pressure slowly and diligently into the tissue at an oblique angle using your hand, a loose fist, the heel of your hand and even your elbow followed by waiting for the tissue to yield and permit movement longitudinally, transverse or a combination of both. Like the other MFR techniques already mentioned, myofascial mobilisations use no lubrication because the greatest benefit from the technique is to wait for the tissue to permit movement without sliding or gliding over the skin. Many therapists describe these techniques as a gliding *through* the tissues, and it is important to note that this sensation of moving through the tissues is generated by the feeling of the tissues softening. Don't be tempted to push and force the tissue. There is a real skill to these techniques, which clients describe as pleasantly painful but greatly beneficial.

The same application mentioned above can also be enhanced with both active and passive movement of the joint. This style is often called a lever or a pin and stretch technique, where a joint is used as a lever to lengthen the tissue being treated. The therapist pins, holds or applies a lock to the tissue with the hand, a loose fist or elbow, and then performs an active or passive movement of a joint acting as a lever.

It is not always necessary to actively or passively move the joint in the range of motion specific to the muscle being treated. This is because the fascia of one muscle is connected to the synergistic muscle and even the antagonist, as mentioned in chapter 1. Additionally, the fascia surrounding muscle and adjacent to it is involved in muscular contraction by expanding the radial circumference of the muscle, thereby bringing the insertion and origin closer together.

Some clients simply can't tolerate firm pressure due to their condition, which may even include sensitivity to touch, called peripheral or central sensitisation. This is where the real benefit of MFR comes in: The approach encompasses so many different methods of treating all of the soft tissues, and all these methods are built on the principle of working slowly and diligently within the client's tolerance. When one style of MFR doesn't suit the client, there is always another way.

Combining Techniques

The MFR approach doesn't have boundaries. Therapists often find that they develop their own style, adapt techniques and even invent their own techniques to meet each client's needs. Unlimited technique styles can be integrated and tweaked by refining hand positions, using therapeutic tools or offering multi-therapist treatments and intensive treatments. In this way, you can offer a totally individualised therapy yet maintain the authenticity of the approach.

Chapter 12 addresses combining and adapting techniques, as well as enhancing your felt sense by using fascial assessment as part of a technique. The concept of MFR is not just to use the same technique for the same amount of time to achieve an expected result. It is about making the therapy your own, creating a style and developing a felt sense. In this chapter you learned how to change, refine and adapt techniques to create your own variations on a theme to suit your needs and those of your clients.

TIP Trust what your hands are telling you. If you feel that you need to perform a cross-hand release somewhere else, do that and see what happens.

Closing Remarks

A discussion of combining techniques can sound quite linear. In fact, it is anything but. MFR is a diverse and fluid therapy incorporating relevant techniques derived from the felt sense, what you feel happening under your hands and via your own intuition and feedback from the client.

You may start your treatment with an arm pull and then moments later become drawn from client feedback and tissue change to perform a cross-hand release over the pectoral area. You may also get feedback that the client is feeling changes distant to where you are working. You may move from a cross-hand release or a myofascial mobilisation to a leg pull.

As you become more experienced with MFR, your hands will intuitively know what they need to do and where they need to be. As I have mentioned, the techniques are the instrument; it's how you play the instrument that makes the music.

TIP Practise one technique at a time and become comfortable with it before you try another. Some therapists find incorporating MFR into their existing practices a challenge. Either promote MFR as a separate treatment or ask permission from existing clients to use MFR for 15 minutes at the beginning of the session. Even better, attend a course or get some MFR treatment yourself to help you with these techniques.

As your skill with the MFR approach develops, you will have questions and want to understand what is happening as you work. Your client may also ask you to provide answers and try to make sense of their physical and emotional responses to the treatment.

Learn to trust your intuition and to follow your felt sense. Eventually, questions become unimportant, and you will begin to realise the importance of receiving regular treatment yourself. You will learn more about the work by receiving it than doing it. As your experiences unfold, you will be able to turn them into approaches and techniques to benefit others.

Encourage your clients to explore their responses and sensations to your treatments. Keep in mind that it is not your role to counsel or analyse.

Quick Questions

1. Should massage cream, lotion or oil be used with MFR?
2. What is another name for arm and leg pulls?
3. Why should you stay away from analytical questions when performing MFR?
4. In which direction is fascia predominantly aligned?
5. What is the average length of time needed to perform an MFR technique?

PART III

Applying MFR Techniques

This part of the book describes the techniques in the integrated approach to MFR, namely, the cross-hand releases, longitudinal plane releases, transverse plane releases, scar tissue management approaches and myofascial mobilisations. These chapters offer descriptions of how to position your client on the treatment table and how and where to stand or sit to perform the technique to ensure good body mechanics. These descriptions are supported with photographs and tips about what you and your client might feel and see during the process, as well as tips to ensure client safety and comfort.

Cross-Hand Release Approaches

Cross-hand release techniques are performed with your hands pointing in opposite directions. On some body parts and limbs where there simply isn't enough room for your hands to completely point away from each other, and for comfort and good body mechanics, you will need to place your hands in a position as close to opposite as comfortable to apply the technique. Follow the photographs beside each technique, but if your hands are not comfortable, change to a position that works for you.

Every cross-hand technique is applied with the clear intention of connecting with yourself and the client as well as telling the client what you are about to do. When you complete the techniques, look for vasomotor responses or red flare and perform MFR techniques in those areas and in areas where the client experienced effects and sensations.

Read this chapter through first before performing any of the cross-hand techniques. The first technique is described in full, and subsequent descriptions include the positioning, hand placement and any information relevant to them. Practise the cross-hand release technique of the anterior thigh first to learn how to flow with the entire process, and then the subsequent techniques will make more sense.

Cross-Hand Release of the Anterior Thigh

The cross-hand release of the anterior thigh is probably the easiest technique to apply and therefore the best way to get the feel of MFR. Notice that I use the term *anterior thigh* and not *the quadriceps area*. This is because you will be feeling more than the muscle alone. We so often focus on muscle and neglect all of the many other structures and soft tissues that make up the entire structure. When performing MFR, you should focus on the three-dimensional fascial matrix and all that it supports and protects.

   Position your client supine (face up) on your treatment table, with as much of the body uncovered as the client is comfortable with, and remember not to apply any oil, lotion or massage cream. The reason for performing MFR without covering the client with towels, sheets and quilts is that you will be constantly looking for and listening to what is happening in the client's body. If the body is covered, you may miss these things. (See chapter 3 for more information on using equipment and setting the scene.)

1. Stand at the side of the treatment table.
2. Soften your own body, allow yourself to feel comfortable in your own skin and focus on your client's needs.
3. Set an intention to communicate with, help and respond to the client, rather than to what you want to do.
4. Tell the client what you are going to do.
5. Place one flat hand above the kneecap on the soft tissue with the arc of your hand, between your thumb and index finger, cupping the client's kneecap.
6. Place your other hand, with the fingers pointing in the opposite direction, flat onto the client's thigh so that your hands are crossed.
7. Allow both of your hands to soften onto the client's thigh.
8. Ask the client to become aware of where your hands are, and allow the client's body to become soft and receptive to your hands.
9. Lean into the tissue to find the subtle depth barrier of tissue resistance.
10. Wait for the tissue to yield under your hands (a butter-melting sensation), then take up the slack under your hands by gently and slowly leaning into the next depth barrier of tissue resistance. Stop there and wait until you feel the tissue change again and follow it to the next tissue barrier. Remember never to force the tissue; always be gentle.
11. Take notice of the tissue change, and eventually you will begin to feel a yielding of the tissue between your hands as well as a tissue-melting sensation under your hands.
12. Maintain your inward pressure whilst at the same time taking up the slack between your hands (move your hands away from each other without force to the tissue barrier) without slipping or gliding over the skin. Following two dimensions, hold and wait for the tissue to change and soften.

13. Take a look at the client's body and ask them what they are noticing either under your hands or anywhere else in the body.

14. Eventually, you will feel movement in another direction under your hands. This is the third dimension; follow this sensation of tissue change in the same manner as the first two dimensions, again without using force or slipping over the skin.

15. Every time the tissue changes in any direction, take up the available slack and wait at the next barrier of tissue resistance, always maintaining pressure at the depth barrier.

16. Follow the tissues as they soften and yield for approximately three to five minutes or more for optimal results.

17. Once again, ask what the client is noticing occurring in the body.

18. Slowly disengage your hands and look for red flare on the client's body.

19. If the client has experienced sensations, feelings, heat or coolness, or you have noticed red flare, these are areas that require subsequent treatment and may be part of a physical holding pattern.

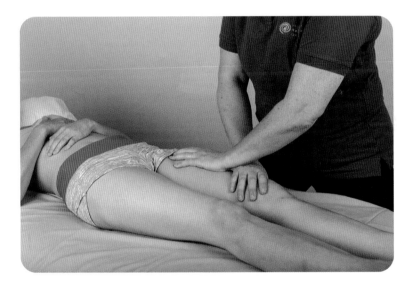

TIP To increase your sense awareness, perform the same technique on the client's other anterior thigh so you can compare the results. You may notice that one leg is different than the other. This in itself can offer valuable information about the client's physical status, which you can then add to your palpatory assessment findings.

Cross-Hand Release of the Anterior Lower Leg

Because the anterior lower leg has so much less soft tissue than the anterior thigh does, even though the process of the cross-hand released technique is the same, you will feel the difference of the tissue composition in that the bone offers more resistance under your hands.

1. Have the client lie supine on the treatment table with the leg straight.
2. Stand at the side of the treatment table.
3. Place one hand, skin on skin, on the client's anterior lower leg close to the ankle with the arc of your hand between the thumb and index finger cupping the anterior ankle and your fingers wrapping around the medial ankle.
4. Place your other hand just below the client's knee, cupping the inferior aspect of the kneecap with the arc of your hand between your thumb and index finger.
5. Lean into the client to the tissue depth barrier, wait and follow the subtle three-dimensional changes in the tissue.
6. Avoid forcing the tissue or slipping or gliding over the skin.
7. Apply the technique for at least three to five minutes for optimal results.

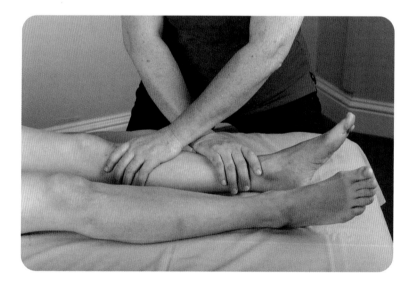

Cross-Hand Release of the Medial Arch of the Foot

This technique addresses not only the plantar fascia but also the entire length of the fascia from the foot upwards and can make a huge difference to how the foot functions.

1. Have the client lie supine on the treatment table with the leg straight and slightly externally rotated and supported as required, taking care to protect the knee joint.
2. Sit at the bottom end of the treatment table.
3. Place one hand, skin on skin, on the medioanterior aspect of the foot (head of the first metatarsal), using it as a handle.
4. Place your other hand, skin on skin, on the medial ankle, using the heel bone (calcaneus) as a handle.
5. Lean into the client to the tissue depth barrier, wait and follow the subtle three-dimensional changes in the tissue.
6. Avoid forcing the tissue or slipping or gliding over the skin.
7. Apply the technique for at least three to five minutes for optimal results.

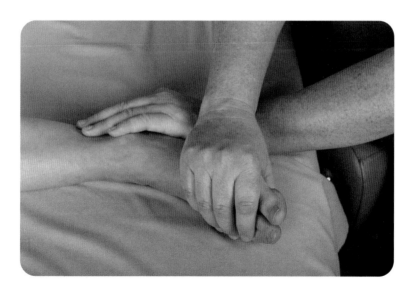

Cross-Hand Release of the Posterior Thigh

Any MFR technique performed on the legs helps keep not just the joints of the knee, hip and foot balanced but the pelvis and the structures superior to it as well.

1. Have the client lie prone on the treatment table with the legs straight.
2. Stand at the side of the treatment table.
3. Place one hand, skin on skin, on the client's posterior thigh close to the back of the knee with your fingers pointing towards the client's ankle or wrapping around the thigh.
4. Place your other hand just below the client's ischial tuberosity, where the hamstring muscles attach, with your fingers pointing towards the client's head.
5. Lean into the client to the tissue depth barrier, wait and follow the subtle three-dimensional changes in the tissue.
6. Avoid forcing the tissue or slipping or gliding over the skin.
7. Apply the technique for at least three to five minutes for optimal results.
8. This technique can be more focused if you place your hand over the ischial tuberosity, using it as a handle.

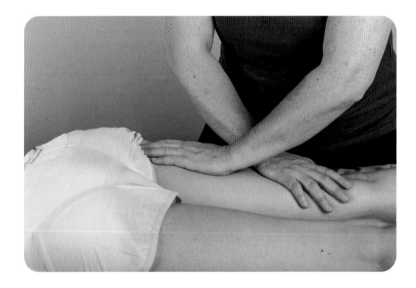

Cross-Hand Release of the Posterior Lower Leg

1. Have the client lie prone on the treatment table with the legs straight and ankles over the end of the treatment table.
2. Stand at the side of the treatment table.
3. Place one hand, skin on skin, on the client's posterior lower leg with the arc of your hand between the thumb and index finger cupping the posterior ankle.
4. Place your other hand just below the client's posterior knee with your fingers pointing towards the client's head.
5. Lean into the client to the tissue depth barrier, wait and follow the subtle three-dimensional changes in the tissue.
6. Avoid forcing the tissue or slipping or gliding over the skin.
7. Apply the technique for at least three to five minutes for optimal results.

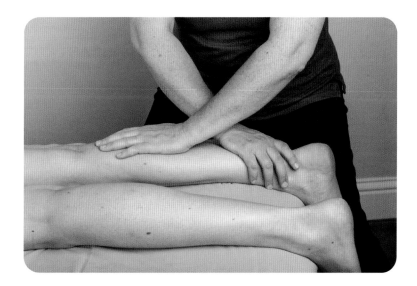

Cross-Hand Release of the Lateral Upper Leg

1. You may find that you have better body mechanics if you stand in front of, rather than behind, the client to perform this technique. Stand on the side of the treatment table that offers better body mechanics for you.
2. Have the client assume a side-lying position with the leg you are working on straight and supported by a pillow or the other leg.
3. Stand at the side of the treatment table in front of the client.
4. Place one hand, skin on skin, on the client's lateral leg just above the knee with your fingers pointing towards the ankle.
5. Place your other hand just below the client's lateral hip with your fingers pointing toward the hip.
6. Lean into the client to the tissue depth barrier, wait and follow the subtle three-dimensional changes in the tissue.
7. Avoid forcing the tissue or slipping or gliding over the skin.
8. Apply the technique for at least three to five minutes for optimal results.

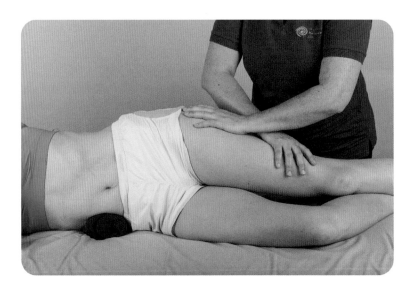

Cross-Hand Release of the Medial Upper Leg

1. Have the client assume a side-lying position with the leg you are working on lying straight on the treatment table and the leg you are not working on in front of the client and supported by a pillow.
2. Stand at the side of the treatment table behind the client.
3. Place one hand, skin on skin, on the client's medial leg just above the knee with your fingers pointing towards the ankle.
4. Place your other hand just below the client's pelvis with your fingers pointing towards the pelvis.
5. Lean into the client to the tissue depth barrier, wait and follow the subtle three-dimensional changes in the tissue.
6. Avoid forcing the tissue or slipping or gliding over the skin.
7. Apply the technique for at least three to five minutes for optimal results.
8. Working in this area can be very beneficial for pelvic balancing because of the structures that attach to the pubic area.
9. Make sure the client doesn't roll forwards, and has adequate support under the top leg; otherwise, there will not be enough room for your hands.

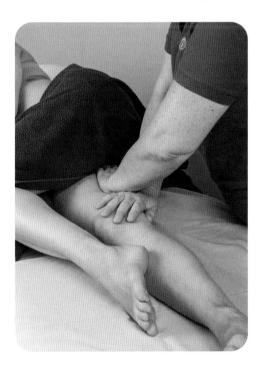

Cross-Hand Release of the Upper Arm

1. Have the client lie supine on the treatment table with the arm straight and externally rotated at the shoulder joint and with the palm of the hand facing upwards.

2. Stand at the side of the treatment table.

3. Place one hand, skin on skin, on the client's upper arm with your hand contacting the shoulder joint, fingers pointing towards the client's head.

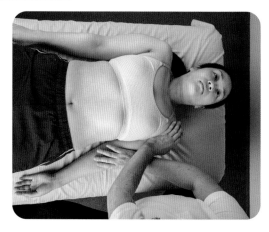

4. Place your other hand just above the client's elbow with your fingers pointing towards the client's wrist.

5. Lean into the client to the tissue depth barrier, wait and follow the subtle three-dimensional changes in the tissue.

6. Avoid forcing the tissue or slipping or gliding over the skin.

7. Apply the technique for at least three to five minutes for optimal results.

Cross-Hand Release of the Elbow Joint

1. Have the client lie supine on the treatment table with the arm to be treated straight and externally rotated at the shoulder joint and with the palm of the hand facing upwards.

2. Stand at the side of the treatment table.

3. Place one hand, skin on skin, on the client's upper arm with your fingers pointing towards the client's head.

4. Place your other hand just below the client's elbow with your fingers pointing towards the wrist.

5. Lean into the client to the tissue depth barrier, wait and follow the subtle three-dimensional changes in the tissue.

6. Avoid forcing the tissue or slipping or gliding over the skin.

7. Apply the technique for at least three to five minutes for optimal results.

Cross-Hand Release of the Upper Chest (Pectoralis Area)

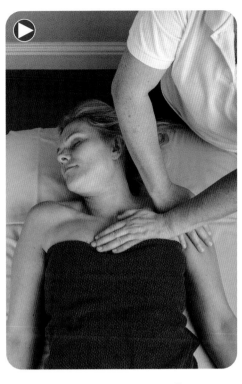

1. Have the client lie supine on the treatment table without a pillow, with the arm and wrist you are working on straight and externally rotated at the shoulder joint and with the palm of the hand facing upwards. Rotate the client's head and neck away from the side you are treating.

2. Stand at the top corner or the side of the treatment table depending on where you feel comfortable.

3. Place one hand, skin on skin, on the client's anterior shoulder joint with your fingers pointing towards the client's wrist and slightly lateral to contour their arm.

4. Place your other hand slightly lateral to the sternum of the side you are working on with your fingers over the sternum and pointing towards the opposite axilla.

5. Lean into the client to the tissue depth barrier, wait and follow the subtle three-dimensional changes in the tissue.

6. Avoid forcing the tissue or slipping or gliding over the skin.

7. Apply the technique for at least three to five minutes for optimal results.

TIP This is a great technique for the chest and can help with upper back and shoulder issues. To maximise the benefit of this technique, perform it on both sides of the chest.

Cross-Hand Release of the Anterior Hip

1. Have the client lie supine on the treatment table with the legs straight.

2. Stand at the side of the treatment table.

3. Place one hand, skin on skin, on the client's lower abdominal area just above the anterior superior iliac spine (ASIS) with your fingers pointing towards the opposite shoulder.

4. Place your other hand on the upper thigh just below the ASIS with your fingers pointing towards the client's feet.

5. Lean into the client to the tissue depth barrier, wait and follow the subtle three-dimensional changes in the tissue.

6. Avoid forcing the tissue or slipping or gliding over the skin.

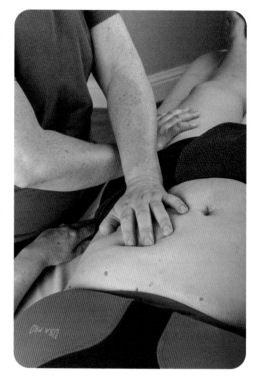

7. Apply the technique for at least three to five minutes for optimal results.

TIP
- Remember that no abdominal MFR may be performed on ladies who are pregnant.
- This technique often elicits what we describe as a therapeutic burn or stinging sensation, which is a normal response to tissue change.

CLIENT TALK

I often use this technique for clients with low back, sacral and sciatic issues.

Cross-Hand Release of the Anterior Thigh and Anteriorly Rotated Ilium

This technique, which assists with pelvic balancing, is almost identical to the first cross-hand release technique in this chapter, although the position of one hand is much more specific so that you can use the technique to address an anteriorly rotated ilium.

To see and feel how this technique works, you need to locate and take note of four bony landmarks on the client's body: the two anterior superior iliac spines (ASIS) and the two posterior superior iliac spines (PSIS). See chapter 4 for how to locate these.

The following pelvic assessment is helpful to perform before doing the cross-hand release of anterior rotated ilium.

Palpatory Pelvic Assessment

1. Ask the client, who is supine on the treatment table, to bend the knees and bring the feet together, close to the buttocks.

2. Ask the client to lift the hips off the treatment table and then to rest them back down and straighten the legs. This gives you the opportunity to visually assess any pelvic imbalance because the client is out of gravity thereby eliminating compensatory patterns.

3. Ask the client to straighten the legs.

4. Stand at the foot of the treatment table and bring the client's ankles close together and notice the level of the medial ankle bones (malleoli). Very often one ankle bone looks lower than (inferior to) the other.

5. Next, stand to the side of the client's hips and place your flat hands over both ASIS.

6. Using your thumbs as markers, hook under both ASIS and notice which one looks lower than (inferior to) the other.

Often, the ankle bone that looks lower (inferior) is on the same side as the ASIS that looks lower (inferior). This is called a pelvic imbalance and a leg length discrepancy. This is a very simplistic assessment, but if you perform the following technique on the side where the ASIS looked lower (inferior) and then retest by asking the client to raise the hips again, you may see a significant result.

Cross-Hand Release to Balance the Pelvis

1. Have the client lie supine on the treatment table with the legs straight.

2. Stand at the side of the treatment table, on the side where the client's ASIS is lower (inferior).

3. Place one hand, skin on skin, over the client's ASIS, using it as a handle with your fingers pointing towards the client's head.

4. Place your other hand on the upper thigh just below the ASIS with fingers pointing towards the feet.

5. Lean into the client to the tissue depth barrier, wait and follow the subtle three-dimensional changes in the tissue.

6. Avoid forcing the tissue or slipping or gliding over the skin.

7. Apply the technique for at least three to five minutes for optimal results.

8. As the tissue changes, you will begin to feel the ilia posteriorly rotate or tilt.

9. Follow the tissues as they change, encouraging the ilia to move, as you apply your subtle pressure to the ASIS and recheck the bony landmarks when you have completed the technique.

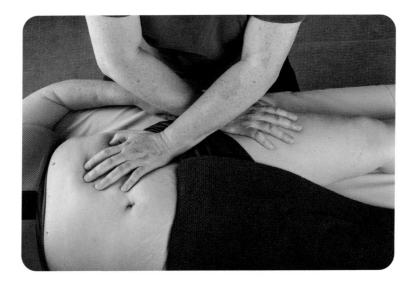

Cross-Hand Release of the Lumbosacral Junction (L5-S1 Decompression)

1. Have the client lie prone on the treatment table with the legs straight.
2. Stand at the side of the treatment table.
3. Place one hand, skin on skin, on the client's sacrum with the arc of your hand across the sacrum and clearing the buttock cleft.
4. Place your other hand on the lower lumbar spine with fingers pointing towards the client's head.
5. Lean into the client to the tissue depth barrier, wait and follow the subtle three-dimensional changes in the tissue.
6. Avoid forcing the tissue or slipping or gliding over the skin.
7. Apply the technique for at least three to five minutes for optimal results.

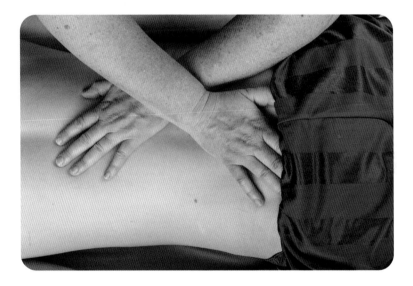

CLIENT TALK

Many people struggle with compressed discs as well as lumbar and sacral pain and dysfunction. This is an effective technique for relieving the tension in this area.

Cross-Hand Release of the Upper Back

1. Have the client lie prone on the treatment table.
2. Stand at the top of the treatment table.
3. Place the palm of your hand, skin on skin, lateral to the spine with your fingers lying across the medial border of the scapula and onto the scapula.
4. Place your other hand in the same place on the opposite side.
5. Lean into the client to the tissue depth barrier, wait and follow the subtle three-dimensional changes in the tissue.
6. Avoid forcing the tissue or slipping or gliding over the skin.
7. Apply the technique for at least three to five minutes for optimal results.

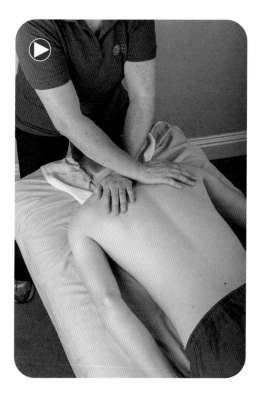

TIP This technique can also be performed with one hand on the client's upper back and the other hand on the client's low back on the same side or on a diagonal.

Cross-Hand Release of the Lateral Low Back Area

1. Have the client lie diagonally across the treatment table with the top leg straight and positioned slightly behind the body and over the edge of the treatment table.
2. Place a small pillow or rolled-up towel beneath the client's waist to keep the lumbar spine neutral.
3. If possible, have the client place the top arm over their head (or as far in front as possible) to maximise the entire lengthening of the body.
4. Stand at the side of the treatment table behind the client.
5. Place one hand, skin on skin, over the iliac crest, using it as a handle, with your fingers pointing towards the client's feet.
6. With fingers pointing towards the client's head, place your other hand over the lower ribs and soft tissue between the ribs and hips.
7. Lean into the client to the tissue depth barrier, wait and follow the subtle three-dimensional changes in the tissue.
8. Avoid forcing the tissue or slipping or gliding over the skin.
9. Apply the technique for at least three to five minutes for optimal results.
10. Lift the client's arm and leg back to the midline after completing this technique.

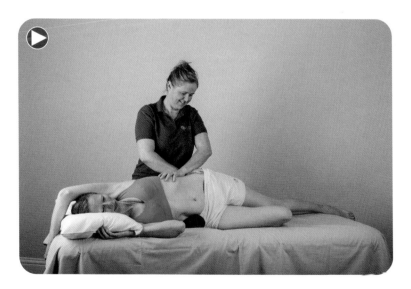

TIP Although this technique is great for general back issues, take care with positioning for any client who has disc or nerve issues. Cease the technique if the client begins to experience nerve pain, and instead perform the technique with the client in the prone position.

Cross-Hand Release of the Lateral Hip

1. Have the client lie diagonally across the treatment table with the top leg straight and positioned slightly behind the body and over the edge of the table.

2. Place a small pillow or rolled-up towel beneath the waist to keep the lumbar spine neutral.

3. If possible, have the client place the top arm over their head (or as far in front of the body as possible) to maximise the entire lengthening of the lateral tissue.

4. Stand at the side of the treatment table behind the client.

5. Place one hand, skin on skin, on the upper lateral thigh with your fingers pointing toward the client's feet.

6. With your fingers pointing towards the client's head, place your other hand slightly inferior to the iliac crest.

7. Lean into the client to the tissue depth barrier, wait and follow the subtle three-dimensional changes in the tissue.

8. Avoid forcing the tissue or slipping or gliding over the skin.

9. Apply the technique for at least three to five minutes for optimal results.

10. Lift the client's arm and leg back to the midline after completing this technique.

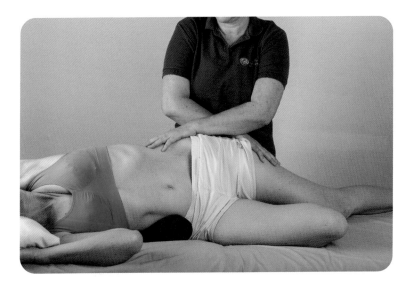

TIP Like the lateral low back technique, this technique is great for general back issues; however, take care with the positioning for any client who has disc or nerve issues. Cease the technique if the client begins to experience nerve pain, and instead perform the technique with the client in the prone position.

This is one of my favourite techniques because it helps clients with low back issues, pelvic imbalances and leg length discrepancies.

Cross-Hand Release of the Lateral Neck and Shoulder, Side Lying

1. Have the client assume a side-lying position, without a pillow, on the treatment table with the upper arm lying on the side of the body.

2. Stand or sit at the top, or top corner, of the treatment table, whichever is more comfortable.

3. Place one hand, skin on skin, on the anterolateral shoulder, using the shoulder joint as a handle, with your fingers pointing towards the client's hips.

4. Place your other hand, skin on skin, on the lateral side of the neck and face. If you have your hands crossed, as in the first photo, your fingers will point towards the client's head. If you have not crossed your hands, as in the second photo, your fingers will point towards the client's feet.

5. Lean into the client to the tissue depth barrier, wait and follow the subtle three-dimensional changes in the tissue.

6. Avoid forcing the tissue or slipping or gliding over the skin.

7. Apply the technique for at least three to five minutes for optimal results.

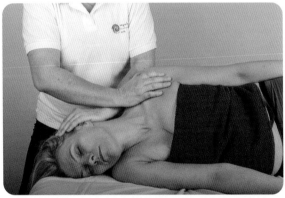

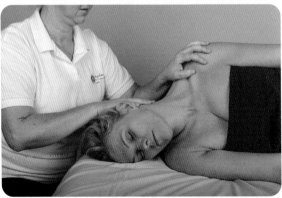

TIP Take care with the positioning for any client who has disc or nerve issues. Cease the technique if the client begins to experience nerve pain, and instead perform the technique with the client in a supine position. For this technique you do not necessarily need to cross your hands; however, the application is the same as any other cross-hand release technique.

Cross-Hand Release of the Anterior Cervical Spine

Although this technique is considered a cross-hand release technique, it is slightly different to the others because it is performed through the body and specifically the cervical spine, treating the structures of the suboccipital area and the cervical spine.

The hand that supports the head and neck waits for the head to soften into it and for the neck to lengthen, and takes up the slack with any tissue softening to the next barrier of resistance. At the same time, the top hand sinks into the chest and sternal area waiting for a yielding sensation in both an inward and inferior direction (towards the feet). The sensation of tissue softening is followed through each barrier in the same way as any other cross-hand release.

1. Have the client lie supine on the treatment table with no pillow.
2. Sit at the top of the treatment table.
3. Support the client's head with one hand, either with your fingers pointing towards the feet or with your fingers pointing to one of the shoulders, whichever is more comfortable for your wrist.
4. Place your other hand, skin on skin, on the client's chest with your palm contacting the sternum and your fingers pointing towards the client's feet.
5. Allow the client's head to soften into your supporting hand whilst the top hand sinks inwards to the depth barrier of tissue resistance. Wait and follow the subtle yielding of the tissue.
6. As the client's neck softens, gently draw the client's head and neck towards you whilst applying a gentle pressure towards the feet with your top hand.
7. Continue through each barrier until a significant softening of the tissue has occurred.
8. Always wait at the tissue barrier, never forcing the tissue or slipping or gliding over the skin.
9. Apply the technique for at least three to five minutes for optimal results.

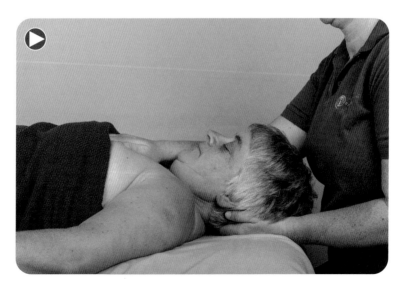

Closing Remarks

Many people who have learned MFR have been taught to either stretch the tissue initially and then wait for the tissue to change or unwind using light pressure of around 0.18 ounces (5 g). Although this may be correct for other types of body-work, in MFR we meet, follow and facilitate any tissue changes as opposed to forcing it or staying only at the elastin barrier.

This chapter describes specific cross-hand releases. However, once you understand the concept of the technique, cross-hand releases can be applied anywhere on the body.

Remember that MFR is not a symptomatic therapy; in other words, it does not focus on treating symptoms. Symptoms may arise in one area of the body but could be a result of a restriction elsewhere within the three-dimensional fascial matrix. For this reason, there are no specific techniques for specific aches, pains and injuries. The entire fascial matrix must be treated to remove the tensional forces on pain-receptive structures.

Make sure to check your body mechanics before starting each technique. When you are standing, keep your back straight and your head up and slightly posteriorly rotated; tilt your pelvis to protect your low back. Keep your arms close to your body and allow your elbows and wrists to be soft and relaxed. If you feel your body begin to fatigue, it is OK to move or re-place your hands, but you must start the technique from the beginning again.

Practice makes perfect. Cross-hand release techniques are a great way to begin your MFR therapy journey because they build confidence and intuition and enhance the development of a kinaesthetic felt sense awareness.

Quick Questions

1. Are cross-hand release techniques just for treating muscles?
2. What must you be careful of when performing the lateral lumbar release technique?
3. Can you perform abdominal MFR on pregnant ladies?
4. What bony landmark at the front of the pelvis do you place your hand on when you want to de-rotate the ilia?
5. Do we use oil or lotion to perform cross-hand release techniques?

Longitudinal Plane Releases

Longitudinal plane releases derive their name from the fact that the techniques treat the fascia and its associated structures throughout the length of the body. Because fascia is predominantly aligned top to toe, longitudinal plane releases, or arm and leg pulls, are an excellent way of lengthening and realigning the body.

As in the majority of the cross-hand release techniques, you will perform arm and leg pulls whilst you are standing. As you lean back ever so slightly to take up the slack, or traction, in the limb, you create a counterbalance with your body weight. This counterbalance must be precise, because overpulling or creating too much traction will cause the client to tense and the technique to become harder to perform, if not useless. Always remember that less is more.

Positioning the client and performing the arm and leg pulls at a variety of angles maximise the results of the technique. In general, the intention of performing an arm or leg pull is to treat the entire structure of the limb, which includes the associated joints and any structures within the line of pull through to the opposite side and other end of the body. These techniques can also include circumduction of the shoulder and hip joints to facilitate a greater tissue change.

For the purpose of teaching, I describe some of the techniques as beginning with traction followed first by external rotation and then by abduction. As you become more experienced, you will notice that the techniques become more fluid and less linear. Ultimately, as long as you are working in three dimensions, or planes of movement, you can perform these positions in any order.

With all of the techniques in this chapter, set an intention before the treatment to engage with yourself and your client (focusing, or grounding, followed by connection), tell the client what you're going to do and dialogue with the client during the treatment so you can learn of any responses and effects being experienced. Also, when you complete the techniques, look for vasomotor responses, or red flare. Perform MFR techniques in those areas and anywhere the client experienced effects and sensations from the longitudinal plane release.

As with the cross-hand release techniques, the first longitudinal plane release technique in this chapter is described in detail; descriptions of subsequent techniques include hand placements and any aspects specific to those techniques. I suggest you read this entire chapter before performing the techniques because it will help you become more fluid with them and enhance your felt sense awareness.

Arm Pull Supine

1. Have the client lie supine on the treatment table with no pillow.

2. Practise the movement of the arm first without employing the fascial element so that you can practise your hand positions. This might help you with the full circumduction.

3. Stand at the side of the treatment table.

4. Gently hold the client's lower arm with both hands in a position that is comfortable for you; do not grasp the client's wrist. Lift the arm gently off the treatment table so that your back and shoulders are comfortable.

5. Gently traction the arm by leaning back slightly until you feel a subtle resistance and the tissue end-feel; do not force the barrier or slip over the skin.

6. Whilst maintaining the traction phase, externally rotate the arm at the shoulder joint until you meet resistance and the tissue end-feel without forcing the barrier.

7. Whilst maintaining the first two dimensions, abduct the arm away from the body until you meet resistance and the tissue end-feel again without forcing the barrier.

8. Maintain these three barriers, waiting for any one of them to soften, at which point you take up the slack to the next tissue barrier, or end-feel, and continue following each yielding sensation.

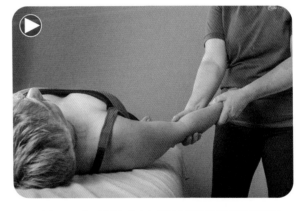

9. As the tissues change in the arm, the arm will move further into abduction and external rotation and will also begin to elongate.

10. Dialogue with the client about any effects of and responses to the treatment.

11. Eventually, the client's arm will be positioned above the head. Maintain the traction on the arm and wait for a further yielding sensation; the arm should now be pointing to the ceiling. Move around the top of the treatment table to the opposite side, bringing the arm with you.

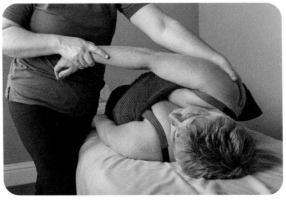

12. Traction the arm to tissue resistance across the body, gently pulling the shoulder towards you. Reach around the lateral shoulder with your other hand, place it on the medial border of the scapula and glide it towards you by leaning backwards.

13. Maintain the traction until you feel an elongation of the entire arm and shoulder, and then gently release the scapula, allowing the client's shoulder to drop back onto the treatment table whilst maintaining the traction on the arm with one hand.

14. Continue tractioning the arm towards the ceiling and walk back around to the opposite side of the treatment table, adducting the arm back to the side.

15. Always perform the technique for at least three to five minutes without forcing the tissue.

CLIENT TALK

Although this technique is great for clients with shoulder problems such as frozen shoulder, rotator cuff injuries and tendinitis (tendinopathy), be aware that these clients will have limited abduction and will not be able to tolerate the full circumduction phase of this technique. In such cases, the arm pull can still offer excellent results by taking the three planes of movement to the available barriers offered by the client.

Leg Pull Supine

1. Have the client lie supine on the treatment table.

2. Stand at the side and towards the lower end of the treatment table.

3. Gently hold the client's lower leg with both hands in a position that is comfortable for you. Lift the leg gently off the treatment table so that your back and shoulders are comfortable; use one of your hands to dorsiflex the ankle if possible.

4. Gently traction the leg by leaning back slightly until you feel a subtle resistance at the tissue end-feel.

5. Whilst maintaining the traction phase, externally rotate the leg at the hip joint until you meet resistance and the tissue end-feel.

6. Whilst maintaining the first two dimensions, abduct they leg away from the body until you meet resistance and the tissue end-feel.

7. Maintain these three barriers, waiting for any one of them to soften. Follow the softening sensation by taking up the available slack to the next tissue barrier; continue following the tissue as it softens.

8. As the leg softens, it will move further into abduction and external rotation and will also begin to elongate.

9. Dialogue with the client about any effects of and responses to the treatment, and check that the knee is comfortable.

10. Eventually, the client's leg will not be able to abduct any farther. Maintaining the traction, lift the leg slowly towards the ceiling, adducting it and moving into hip flexion as you wait for a sense of tissue softening. Move around the bottom of the treatment table to the opposite side, bringing the leg with you; it should now begin to internally rotate.

11. Traction the leg across the body and, gently pulling the hip towards you, place one of your hands on the lateral hip, gliding it towards you. Maintain the leg traction with your other hand; stand below the leg to do this.

12. Maintain the traction until you feel an elongation of the entire leg and hip, and then gently release the hip, allowing it to drop back onto the treatment table whilst maintaining the traction on the leg with one hand.

13. Continue tractioning the leg and gently move it back into hip flexion, walking around to the opposite side of the treatment table and adducting the leg to the side.

14. Remember never to force the barrier in any direction or to slip over the skin. Always perform the technique for a minimum of five minutes, sometimes longer, for optimal results.

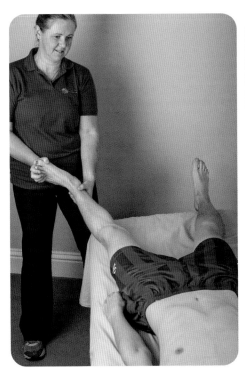 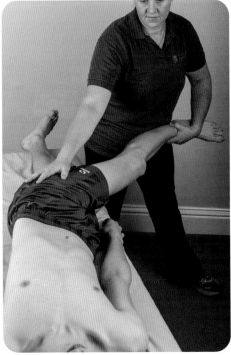

TIP You may wish to practise the leg movements and hand positions for this technique prior to adding the fascial component.

Elbow Pull Supine

1. Have the client lie supine on the treatment table.
2. Stand at the top of the treatment table.
3. Gently hold the client's arm and raise it above the head into shoulder flexion, allowing the elbow to bend.
4. Wrap your fingers around the crease of the client's bent elbow with your thumbs on the posterior elbow.
5. Lift the elbow slightly to the ceiling and to resistance, and at the same time traction the elbow and arm towards you to resistance by leaning back slightly.
6. Dialogue with the client about any effects of and responses to the treatment.
7. Maintain the traction until you feel an elongation of the entire arm and shoulder.
8. Remember never to force the barrier in any direction or to slip over the skin. Always perform the technique for a minimum of five minutes, sometimes longer, for optimal results.

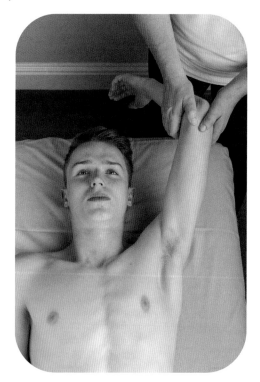

Arm Pull Prone

1. Have the client lie prone on the treatment table.

2. Stand at the side of the treatment table.

3. Gently hold the client's lower arm with both hands in a position that is comfortable for you; do not grasp the client's wrist. Lift the arm gently off the treatment table so that your back and shoulders are comfortable.

4. Gently traction the arm by leaning back slightly until you feel a subtle resistance and the tissue end-feel.

5. Whilst maintaining the traction phase, externally rotate the arm at the shoulder joint until you meet resistance and the tissue end-feel.

6. Whilst maintaining the first two dimensions, abduct the arm away from the body until you meet resistance and the tissue end-feel.

7. Maintain these three barriers, waiting for any one of them to soften, at which point you take up the slack to the next barrier and continue following the tissue as it softens.

8. As the arm softens, it will move further into abduction and external rotation and will also begin to elongate. Move with the arm to the top of the treatment table as the arm softens into shoulder flexion.

9. Dialogue with the client about any effects of and responses to the treatment.

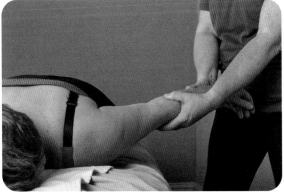

10. Maintain the traction until you feel an elongation of the entire arm and shoulder, then slowly begin to adduct the arm back to the client's side.

11. Remember never to force the barrier in any direction or to slip over the skin. Always perform the technique for a minimum of five minutes, sometimes longer, for optimal results.

CLIENT TALK

This is another effective technique for shoulder and arm issues; however, as in the supine arm pull, clients with certain shoulder problems may not be able to have the arm in shoulder flexion. Stay within the client's available positioning, and you will notice that each time you perform this technique, you will be able to take the arm into a greater range of movement as the restrictions yield.

Leg Pull Prone

1. Have the client lie prone close to the edge of the treatment table of the side you are working on. The feet and ankles should be over the end of the table and the head should be turned to the side.

2. Stand at the side and towards the lower end of the treatment table.

3. Gently hold the client's lower leg with both hands in a position that is comfortable for you, and lift it gently off the treatment table in such a way that your back and shoulders are comfortable. Use one of your hands to dorsiflex the ankle if possible.

4. Gently traction the leg by leaning back slightly until you feel a subtle resistance and the tissue end-feel.

5. Whilst maintaining the traction phase, externally rotate the leg at the hip joint until you meet resistance and the tissue end-feel.

6. Whilst maintaining the first two dimensions, abduct the leg away from the body until you meet resistance and the tissue end-feel.

7. Maintain these three barriers, waiting for any one of them to soften, at which point you take up the slack to the next barrier and continue following any tissue change.

8. As the leg softens, it will move further into abduction and external rotation and will also begin to elongate.

9. Dialogue with the client about any effects of and responses to the treatment, and check that the knee is comfortable.

10. Maintain the traction until you feel an elongation of the entire leg and hip.

11. Continue tractioning the leg, and gently move it back to the midline by adducting it.

12. Remember never to force the barrier in any direction or to slip over the skin. Always perform the technique for a minimum of five minutes, sometimes longer, for optimal results.

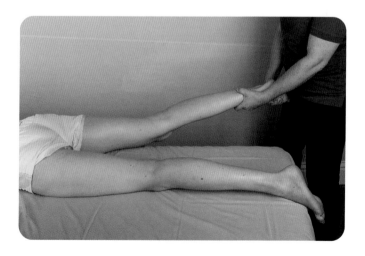

Bilateral Arm Pulls, Prone and Supine

Regardless of whether the client is lying prone or supine, essentially these techniques are identical. The difference in the effect of the technique is in the resultant line of pull, or traction, through the body; basically, you can target specific tissues with appropriate client positioning. This technique is also an effective assessment tool for feeling the differences and similarities of the fascial drag between both sides of the body.

1. Have the client lie prone or supine on the treatment table.
2. Stand at the top of the treatment table.
3. Help the client bring the arm above the head.
4. Gently hold the client's lower arms just above the wrists, or closer to the elbows if the client finds this more comfortable.
5. Gently traction the arms by leaning back slightly until you feel a subtle resistance and the tissue end-feel; the arms will naturally move into slight internal rotation.
6. Dialogue with the client about any effects of and responses to the treatment.
7. Maintain the traction until you feel an elongation of the entire arm and shoulder bilaterally, then slowly replace the arms back to the client's sides.
8. Remember never to force the barrier in any direction or to slip over the skin. Always perform the technique for a minimum of five minutes, sometimes longer, for optimal results.

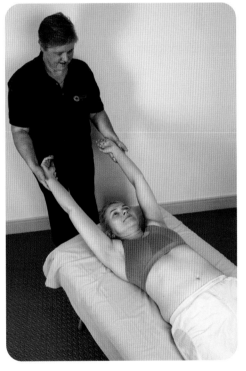

CLIENT TALK

When you traction both arms together, the resultant tissue change will continue all the way down through the body, provided you hold the technique long enough. Clients often report feeling the entire back and pelvis soften during this technique. Stay within the client's available positioning, and always stay at the fascial barrier.

Bilateral Leg Pulls, Prone and Supine

Like the bilateral arm pull, the bilateral leg pull is performed in the same manner in the prone and supine positions. When you traction both legs together, the resultant softening offers an effective treatment throughout the entire body and, in particular, the pelvis and sacrum.

1. Have the client lie prone or supine on the treatment table.
2. Stand at the bottom end of the treatment table.
3. Gently hold the client's lower legs around or just above the ankles, and lift them both gently off the treatment table so that your back and shoulders are comfortable.
4. Gently traction the legs by leaning back slightly until you feel a subtle resistance and the tissue end-feel.
5. Dialogue with the client about any effects of and responses to the treatment.
6. Maintain the traction until you feel an elongation of the entire leg and hip bilaterally.
7. Place the client's legs slowly back onto the treatment table once you have felt a significant elongation and general softening of the tissue.
8. Remember never to force the barrier in any direction or to slip over the skin. Always perform the technique for a minimum of three to five minutes, sometimes longer, for optimal results.

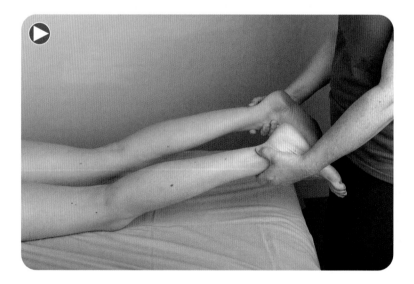

TIP Like the arm pull, this technique is also an effective assessment tool for feeling the differences and similarities of the fascial drag between both sides of the body.

Oppositional Arm and Leg Pulls, Prone and Supine

The human body is constantly trying to compensate for dysfunction and gravity. A common example is a right hip and a left shoulder harbouring dysfunction. In general, where you find contracted tissue (i.e., unable to lengthen), you will also find oppositional tissue (i.e., lengthened, strained and unable to contract). Both contracted and oppositional tissue must be treated to promote balance. Oppositional techniques can help. This technique can be performed by one therapist, using careful client positioning, or by two therapists, as shown in the photo.

1. Have the client lie prone or supine on the treatment table.
2. Stand at the top or bottom corner of the treatment table. If performing this technique with another therapist, the second therapist stands at the diagonally opposite corner of the table.
3. Place one of the limbs into abduction to the end-feel at the barrier of tissue resistance and allow it to rest comfortably on the treatment table and over the edge.
4. Gently hold the client's diagonal opposite limb with your hands in the position for either the arm or leg pull technique, lifting the limb slightly off the treatment table while making sure your back and shoulders remain comfortable.
5. Gently traction the limb by leaning back slightly until you feel a subtle resistance and the tissue end-feel. The limb will naturally fall into internal or external rotation depending on its position of ease.

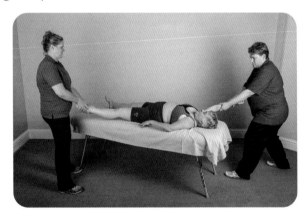

6. Dialogue with the client about any effects of and responses to the treatment.
7. Maintain the traction until you feel an elongation of the entire limb and a sensation of traction towards the opposite diagonal limb.
8. Replace the limbs slowly back onto the treatment table once you have felt a significant elongation and general softening of the tissue. Move to the opposite diagonal limb, and repeat the process.
9. Remember never to force the barrier in any direction or to slip over the skin. Always perform the technique for a minimum of five minutes, sometimes longer, for optimal results.

TIP Like the bilateral arm and leg pulls, oppositional pulls are performed in the same manner regardless of whether the client is lying prone or supine. Effective client positioning will facilitate tissue change and provide an opportunity for another therapist to perform a leg pull whilst you perform the opposite arm pull, or vice versa.

Side-Lying Arm and Leg Pulls

Like oppositional arm and leg pulls, side-lying arm and leg pulls can be performed by one therapist with effective client positioning or by two therapists with one tractioning the arm and the other tractioning the leg, as shown in the photo.

1. Have the client lie diagonally across the treatment table with the top leg straight and positioned slightly behind the client and over the edge of the table.

2. Stand at the top or bottom of the treatment table close to the limb with which you will be working. If working with a second therapist, the other therapist should stand at the opposite end of the table.

3. Place a small pillow or rolled-up towel beneath the client's waist to keep the lumbar spine neutral.

4. If possible, have the client place the top arm over the head (or as far in front of the body as possible) to maximise the entire lengthening of the lateral tissue.

5. Lift either the arm or the leg up from the treatment table (the arm will already be in shoulder flexion and the leg will be positioned in slight hip extension), and apply traction to the end-feel and barrier of resistance.

6. Wait for the yielding sensation and an elongation of the limb into the body and along the lateral side. When this happens, take up the slack to the next barrier of resistance and continue following each yielding sensation.

7. Dialogue with the client about any effects of and responses to the treatment.

8. Re-place the limb gently, move to the opposite end of the treatment table and apply gentle traction to the tissue barrier of the same-side limb, waiting for and following any yielding and elongation offered.

9. Remember never to force the barrier in any direction or to slip over the skin. Always perform the technique for a minimum of three to five minutes, sometimes longer, for optimal results.

10. Lift the client's arm and leg back to the midline after completing this technique.

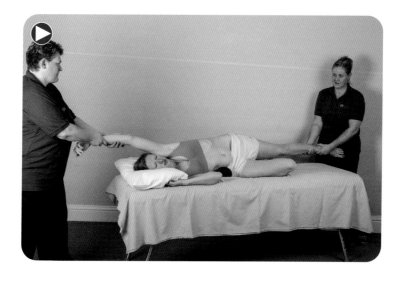

CLIENT TALK

Although this technique is helpful for general back, hip or pelvic issues, take care with the positioning of any client who has disc or nerve issues. Cease the technique if the client begins to experience nerve pain, and instead perform the technique with the client in the prone position.

TIP Arm and leg pulls can take anywhere between 5 and 10 minutes to perform if you include full circumduction of the limb. Make sure to check your body mechanics so that you don't tire when performing these techniques.

Some clients' legs are too heavy to perform a leg pull adequately in the prone or supine position. If you need to rest the leg on the treatment table whilst you perform the technique, you can do so.

Closing Remarks

Longitudinal plane releases are useful as both an assessment tool and technique in their own right. They also work well in combination with the cross-hand release techniques described in chapter 6. It's always an interesting experiment to perform a supine right arm pull followed by a prone right arm pull because it shows how the line of drag and traction affects different structures in different ways.

Arm and leg pulls offer valuable insight into the location of restrictions, increasing kinaesthetic awareness in both therapist and client. Arm and leg pulls will help you feel along the line of traction and notice where that felt sense ends or where the tissue glide comes to a dead halt. Where the tissue feels stuck will be a restriction harbouring dysfunction. Continue to perform an MFR technique in the area that feels stuck, and complete the technique by applying another longitudinal plane technique.

Quick Questions

1. What positions can arm and leg pulls be performed in?
2. What must be placed at the client's lateral low back area when performing a side-lying longitudinal plane release?
3. What must you avoid doing when holding the client's wrist whilst performing an arm pull?
4. What are the three planes, or directions, of movement employed in an arm pull technique?
5. Can you perform full circumduction of the arm in the arm pull technique on a client with a frozen shoulder?

8

Compression Releases

Compression release techniques are techniques in their own right. They are also very useful when cross-hand release techniques or longitudinal plane release techniques fail to provide results because of client discomfort or tissue that is so bound down that it cannot soften and yield.

Restriction binds tissue together, pulling adjacent structures out of alignment and forcing tension onto pain-sensitive areas anywhere in the line of pull. If we apply an MFR technique to these restrictions, eventually the tissue will begin to yield and lengthen. However, sometimes the tissue is so tight, as a result of chronic dysfunction, habitual holding patterns and emotional trauma, that it cannot, or is not ready to, soften and yield. This is where compression techniques come into their own. Because fascia is a three-dimensional tissue, tissue change can be encouraged by waiting for the tissue to soften and yield in any direction including compression. Once the tissue has softened three-dimensionally from performing a compression release technique, subsequent lengthening can be obtained from a cross-hand or longitudinal plane release technique.

As with all MFR techniques, compression techniques are performed skin on skin at the tissue restriction barriers, or end-feel. You lean into, or traction to, the tissue barriers without slipping or gliding over the skin. The tissue should never be forced, and each technique should last for five minutes or more.

TIP Have you ever tried to pull a drawer out of a chest of drawers and found that it simply wouldn't budge? If you push the drawer back in and then pull it out again, the drawer often glides out more easily. This is the concept of compression release techniques: compressing the tissue followed by lengthening it allows it to return to a better range and function.

Essentially, compression release techniques are the opposite of cross-hand release techniques. Instead of crossing your hands, you place your hands side by side, allowing them to sink into the body to the tissue depth barrier of resistance. Then, instead of taking up the slack between your hands by separating them, you allow them to drift closer together to the tissue barrier and then follow any other direction of tissue change offered, through each barrier of resistance.

Like cross-hand release techniques, compression release techniques can be performed anywhere in the body. Following are a few compression release techniques for you to practise; once you get the idea and felt sense of the technique, you can apply the process to any restriction. As in the previous technique chapters, the initial technique is described in full for you to use as a reference when learning all of the ones that follow.

CLIENT TALK

As with all of the other techniques, set your intention and connect with the client in preparing to apply the techniques. Also, don't forget to ask the client for feedback and to check for red flare and responses during and after you have completed the technique.

Compression of the Anterior Thigh

1. Have the client lie supine on the treatment table.
2. Stand at the side of the treatment table.
3. Place both of your hands side by side on the client's anterior thigh.
4. Allow both hands to soften onto the client's thigh.
5. Ask the client to focus on where your hands are and allow the body to become soft and receptive to your hands.
6. Lean into the tissue to find the subtle depth barrier of tissue resistance.
7. Wait for the tissue to yield under your hands (a sensation of butter melting). Then take up the slack under your hands by gently and slowly leaning with your entire body weight into the tissue to the next depth barrier of resistance. Stop there and wait until you feel further tissue change, and follow it.
8. Notice the tissue change. Eventually, you will begin to feel a yielding of the tissue between your hands as well as an inward yielding sensation.
9. Maintain your inward pressure at the depth barrier whilst at the same time taking up the slack between your hands. Compress your hands closer together to meet the tissue resistance as you follow two dimensions; hold and wait for the next yielding sensation.
10. Take your time; don't force the tissue or slip or slide over the skin. Wait approximately three to five minutes or more to allow the tissues to reorganise and soften.
11. Follow this technique in the same manner as a cross-hand release technique, releasing through each barrier three-dimensionally, with the exception of using compression rather than lengthening.
12. Perform a cross-hand release of the same tissues after the compression release.

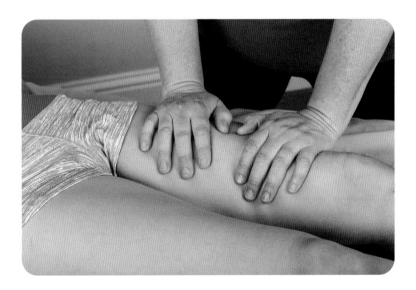

Compression of the Lateral Low Back Area

1. Have the client lie diagonally across the treatment table with the top leg straight and supported by a bolster or pillow.

2. Place a small pillow or rolled-up towel beneath the waist to keep the lumbar spine neutral.

3. If possible, have the client place the top arm over the head (or as far in front as possible) to maximise the lengthening of the lateral tissue.

4. Stand at the side of the treatment table behind the client.

5. Place one hand, skin on skin, over the iliac crest, using it as a handle.

6. Without crossing your hands, place your other hand beside the first hand, slightly inferior to and on the client's lower ribcage.

7. Lean into the tissue to find the subtle depth barrier of tissue resistance.

8. Wait for the tissue to yield under your hands. Then take up the slack under your hands by gently and slowly leaning with your body weight into the tissue to the depth barrier of resistance. Stop there and wait until you feel the tissue soften once more and follow it.

9. Notice the tissue change. Eventually, you will begin to feel a yielding of the tissue between your hands as well as an inward yielding sensation.

10. Maintain your inward pressure to the depth barrier of tissue resistance whilst at the same time taking up the slack between your hands. Compress your hands closer together to meet the tissue barrier as you follow two dimensions; hold and wait for the next yielding sensation.

11. Follow any third dimension offered by taking up the slack to the tissue barrier whilst maintaining the other two dimensions at their tissue barriers.

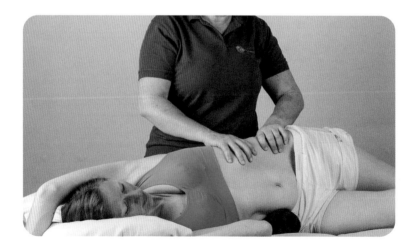

12. Take your time; don't force the tissue or slip or glide over the skin. Wait approximately three to five minutes or more to allow the tissues to reorganise and soften.

13. Follow this technique in the same manner as a cross-hand release technique, releasing through each barrier three-dimensionally, with the exception of using compression rather than lengthening.

14. Perform a cross-hand release of the same tissues after your compression release technique. Move the client's top leg to the edge of the treatment table and slightly over the side of it.

15. Lift the client's arm and leg back to the midline after completing this technique.

CLIENT TALK

Like the cross-hand release technique, this technique is great for general back issues. However, you need to take care with the positioning of any client who has disc or nerve issues. Cease the technique if the client begins to experience nerve pain, and instead perform the technique with the client in the prone position.

Compression of the Posterior Thigh

1. Have the client lie prone on the treatment table with the legs straight.
2. Stand at the side of the treatment table.
3. Place one hand, skin on skin, on the client's posterior thigh close to the back of the knee.
4. Place your other hand beside the first hand just below the client's ischial tuberosity where the hamstring muscles attach.
5. Lean into the tissue to find the subtle depth barrier of tissue resistance.
6. Follow this technique in the same manner as a cross-hand release technique, releasing through each barrier three-dimensionally, with the exception of using compression rather than lengthening at the tissue barrier.
7. Take your time; don't force the tissue or slip or glide over the skin. Wait approximately three to five minutes or more to allow the tissues to reorganise and soften.
8. Perform a cross-hand release of the same tissues after your compression release technique.

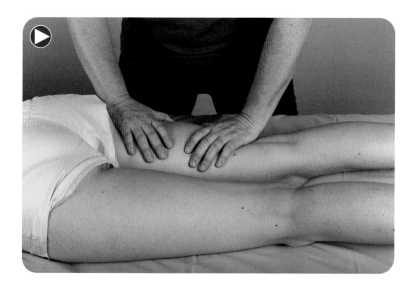

Compression of the Upper Back

1. Have the client lie prone on the treatment table.

2. Stand at the top of the treatment table.

3. Place the palm of one hand, skin on skin, on the scapula close to its medial border. Place your other hand in the same place on the opposite side of the client's back.

4. Lean into the tissue to find the subtle depth barrier of tissue resistance.

5. Follow this technique in the same manner as a cross-hand release technique, releasing through each barrier three-dimensionally, with the exception of using compression rather than lengthening at the tissue barrier.

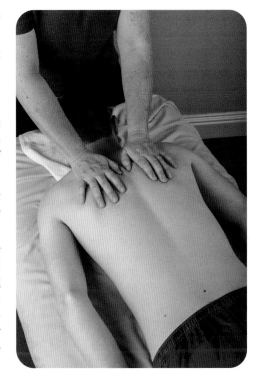

6. Take your time; don't force the tissue or slip or glide over the skin. Wait approximately three to five minutes or more to allow the tissues to reorganise and release.

7. Perform a cross-hand release of the same tissues after your compression technique.

Arm Compression, Prone and Supine

1. Have the client lie supine or prone on the treatment table with no pillow.
2. Stand at the side of the treatment table.
3. Gently hold the client's lower arm with both hands in a position that is comfortable for you; avoid grasping the client's wrist. Lift the arm gently off the treatment table so that your back and shoulders are comfortable.
4. Gently compress the wrist into the elbow, the elbow into the shoulder and the shoulder up into the neck until you feel a subtle resistance and the tissue end-feel.
5. Every time the tissue changes, take up the slack to the next barrier and continue following the tissue as it softens and yields.
6. Once you have obtained significant tissue changes and softening, complete the technique with an arm pull technique as described in chapter 7, which covers longitudinal plane releases.
7. As with all of these techniques, don't force the tissue or slip or glide over the skin. Wait approximately three to five minutes, sometimes more, for optimal results.

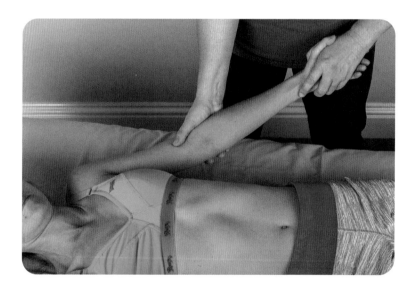

TIP Joint compression release techniques use compression through the associated joints and only slight external rotation following the client's natural positioning. However, you can use compression, external rotation and abduction to enhance the technique.

Essentially, the techniques are identical regardless of whether the client is positioned prone or supine. The difference in the effect of the technique is in the resultant line of compression through the body; you can target specific tissues with appropriate client positioning. These techniques are also effective assessment tools for feeling the differences and similarities of the fascial tension between both sides of the body.

Leg Compression, Prone and Supine

1. Have the client lie supine or prone and slightly towards the edge of the treatment table on the side you are working on, with the feet and ankles over the end of the table.

2. Stand at the side and towards the lower end of the treatment table.

3. Gently hold the client's lower leg with both hands in a position that is comfortable for you. Lift the leg gently off the treatment table so that your back and shoulders are comfortable. Use one of your hands to dorsiflex the ankle if possible.

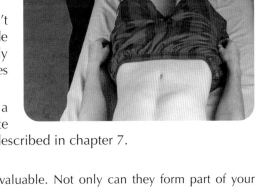

4. Gently compress the ankle into the knee and the knee into the hip until you feel a subtle resistance and the tissue end-feel.

5. Every time the tissue softens, take up the slack to the next barrier and continue following each sensation of softening and tissue change.

6. As with all techniques, don't force the tissue or slip or glide over the skin. Wait approximately three to five minutes, sometimes more, for optimal results.

7. Once you have obtained a significant softening, complete with a leg pull technique as described in chapter 7.

TIP Compression techniques are invaluable. Not only can they form part of your assessment process, but they can also enhance the entire treatment process by binding other techniques together.

As with the longitudinal plane release techniques (arm and leg pulls), make sure that you always facilitate the tissue change to the point at which the client is comfortable; never force the barrier. This is of particular importance for any client with injuries that limit the range of movement. However, repeating the techniques over several sessions will increase this range as well as provide enhanced, pain-free function.

Compression can be used in many ways to resolve restrictions. Some are best combined with other techniques and are beyond the scope of this book. These are learned better in a workshop environment.

Closing Remarks

Compression techniques offer an opportunity to facilitate changes of both physical and emotional constraints hidden deep within the tissue, those that no amount of traction can resolve. Compressed tissue should be treated slowly and subtly, allowing the client to respond naturally in small but significant ways; traction and lengthening of the tissue can simply be too much for some clients to bear.

As in longitudinal plane releases (arm and leg pulls), compression of the joints can be performed unilaterally with the arm or leg placed in any level of abduction from the body. This positioning allows compression of the tissues through the limb, its associated joints and structures, and the rest of the body.

Quick Questions

1. Do you cross your hands when performing a soft tissue compression release technique?
2. Can you perform soft tissue compression release techniques anywhere on the body?
3. Do you perform compression release techniques in a three-dimensional manner?
4. What are the two main client positions for performing compression release techniques of the limbs?
5. Which techniques do you perform after a joint compression release technique?

9

Transverse Plane Releases

The human body has four main transverse planes: the pelvic floor, the respiratory diaphragm, the thoracic inlet and the cranial base. The tissue and fascia in these four areas are denser than the longitudinally oriented fascia because of the role they play in support, balance and structural integrity. The dense nature and positioning of these transverse planes result in any structural imbalance from posture, inflammation and trauma directly influencing their integrity. Moreover, when these areas become tight and restricted, they have a direct effect on the delicate structures above and below them, and in some cases through them, including the internal organs, major blood vessels, lymphatic sites and nerves.

Using MFR techniques, and specifically the transverse plane release techniques, in these regions can create long-lasting reprieves from conditions associated with gastric, urogenital, respiratory and cardiovascular structures; adhesions and scar tissue from surgery; and structural imbalances from injury, trauma, poor posture and inflammation. Transverse plane release techniques can be performed with the client in supine, prone, seated and standing positions. This chapter addresses transverse plane release techniques for the pelvic floor, respiratory diaphragm and thoracic inlet areas; the cranial base release is outside the scope of this book.

When performing transverse plane release techniques, as with all MFR techniques, remember to set an intention to connect with yourself and your clients and to tell your clients what you are going to do before placing your hands on them. Look for red flare and any other responses to the treatment, which will help guide you through the fascial restrictions. Read the entire chapter before performing any techniques to ensure that you understand the hand positions and that your treatments are fluid.

While the joints are not true transverse planes, they provide an articulation of movement on different planes. As such, they become an integration and blending of tissues to support that movement. This means that they do have transverse tissue where transverse plane releases can be effective.

Transverse Plane Release of the Pelvic Floor

1. Have the client lie supine on the treatment table.
2. Sit at the side of the treatment table.
3. Ask the client to bend the knees and lift the hips off the treatment table. Place one hand, skin on skin, under the client's sacrum, with your palm supporting the sacrum and your fingers pointing towards the opposite side. Make sure the thumb of the hand supporting the sacrum is pointing towards the client's head.
4. Place your other hand, skin on skin if possible, directly above your other hand on the client's suprapubic area. It is acceptable to ask the client to place their own hand on the suprapubic area and to rest your hand on top of theirs, again making sure that the thumb of this hand is pointing towards the client's head.
5. Allow the hand beneath the client's sacrum to soften and relax, permitting the client's body weight to rest on it.
6. Ask the client to focus on the area of the body between your hands and allow it to soften and relax.
7. Wait for a sense of yielding of the tissue, and gently allow your top hand to sink inwards to the tissue depth barrier. Follow each sensation of tissue change without slipping or gliding over the skin.
8. Dialogue with the client about any effects of and responses to the technique.
9. Notice the movement under your hand as the tissue yields and softens and follow it in any direction.
10. Perform this technique for at least three to five minutes without forcing the tissue in any direction.

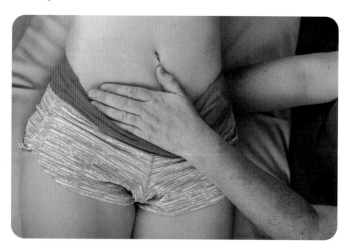

CLIENT TALK

Describe the hand placements of this technique to the client before beginning the treatment, and obtain permission before performing the technique.

Transverse Plane Release of the Respiratory Diaphragm

1. Have the client lie supine on the treatment table.
2. Sit at the side of the treatment table.
3. Ask the client to bend the knees and lift the hips and low back off the treatment table.
4. Place your palm, skin on skin, under the client's thoracolumbar junction area (where T12 meets L5) with your fingers pointing towards the opposite side.
5. Place the palm of your other hand, skin on skin, over the xiphoid process at the end of the client's sternum so that your hand is half on the ribcage and half on the soft tissue.
6. Allow your hand beneath the client to soften and relax, permitting the client's body weight to rest on it.
7. Ask the client to focus on the area of the body between your hands and allow it to soften and relax.
8. Wait for a sense of yielding of the tissue, and gently allow your top hand to sink inwards to the tissue depth barrier. Follow each sensation of tissue change without slipping or gliding over the skin.
9. Dialogue with the client about any effects of and responses to the technique.
10. Notice the movement under your hand as the tissue yields and softens, and follow it in any direction.
11. Perform this technique for at least three to five minutes without forcing the tissue in any direction.

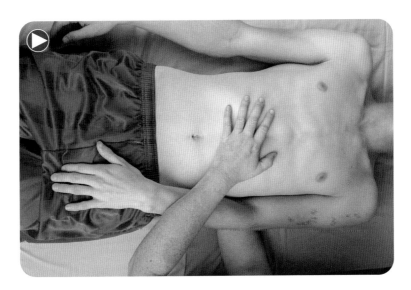

Transverse Plane Release of the Thoracic Inlet, Supine

1. Have the client lie supine on the treatment table.
2. Sit at the side or the corner of the treatment table.
3. Ask the client to lift the upper body off the treatment table so you can place your palm flat, skin on skin, between the shoulder blades at approximately T3 or T4. Make sure that the hand below the client's body is soft and relaxed, allowing the client's body weight to rest on it.
4. Place your other hand, skin on skin, directly above your other hand on the client's upper chest area, below the sternal notch, ensuring that your fingers and thumb are clear of the client's throat.
5. Ask the client to focus on the area of the body between your hands and allow it to soften and relax.
6. Wait for a sense of yielding of the tissue, and gently allow your top hand to sink inwards to the tissue depth barrier. Follow each sensation of tissue change without slipping or gliding over the skin.
7. Dialogue with the client about any effects of and responses to the treatment.
8. Notice the movement under your hand as the tissue yields and softens, and follow it in any direction.
9. Perform this technique for at least three to five minutes without forcing the tissue in any direction.
10. The client can also place their hand on their chest and the therapist places their hand on top of the client's for this technique.

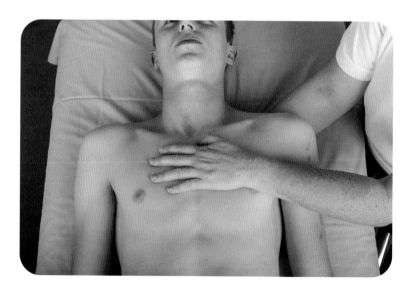

Transverse Plane Release of the Thoracic Inlet, Seated

1. Have the client sit with the back supported and not slouching.
2. Stand to the side of the client.
3. Place your hand, skin on skin, below the sternal notch, ensuring that your fingers and thumb are clear of the client's throat and the sternal notch and that your fingers are pointing away from you.
4. Place your other hand, skin on skin, directly behind your other hand on the client's upper back between the shoulder blades.
5. Ask the client to focus on the area of the body between your hands and allow it to soften and relax.
6. Wait for a sense of yielding of the tissue, and gently allow your top hand to sink inwards to the tissue depth barrier. Follow each sensation of tissue change.

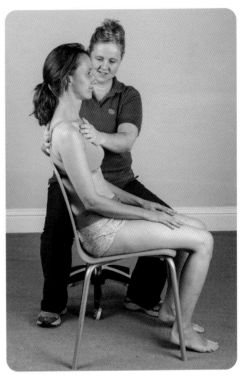

7. Maintaining an inward pressure, engage a downward pressure to the client's hips, waiting for any softening offered without slipping or gliding over the skin.
8. Dialogue with the client about any effects of and responses to the technique.
9. Notice the movement under your hand as the tissue yields and softens, and follow it in any direction.
10. Perform this technique for at least three to five minutes without forcing the tissue in any direction.

Transverse Plane Release of Joints

1. Have the client lie supine or prone on the treatment table.

2. Sit at the side of the treatment table.

3. Place one hand, skin on skin, under the client's joint with the back of your hand resting on the treatment table so that your hand is supporting the joint.

4. Place your other hand, skin on skin, directly above your bottom hand.

5. Allow your hand beneath the client to soften and relax, permitting the weight of the client to rest on it.

6. Ask the client to focus on the area of the body between your hands and allow it to soften and relax.

7. Wait for a sense of yielding of the tissue, and gently allow your top hand to sink inwards to the tissue depth barrier. Follow each sensation of tissue change without slipping or gliding over the skin.

8. Dialogue with the client about any effects of and responses to the treatment.

9. Notice the movement under your hand as the tissue yields and softens, and follow it in any direction.

10. Perform this technique for at least three to five minutes without forcing the tissue in any direction.

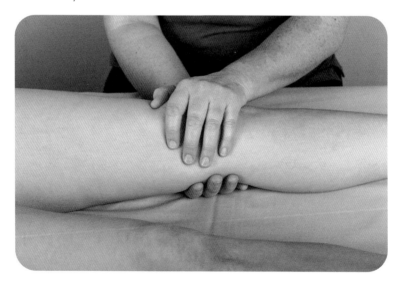

TIP This technique can be performed on any joint of the body using your hands or fingers. When you perform transverse plane release techniques, always make sure that your hand below the client's body remains soft and relaxed so that you can remain tuned in to what you are feeling and following in the client's body.

If the client is uncomfortable about your performing the pelvic floor transverse plane release technique directly, you can perform it through underwear or a sheet. You can obtain a reasonable softening in the tissue through cloth; however, skin-on-skin techniques provide much better results.

Closing Remarks

As with all of the previous MFR techniques, performing transverse plane release techniques in different positions (seated, prone or supine) results in different responses and effects. Some, in particular the thoracic inlet transverse plane release technique, are beneficial for people who cannot lie on the treatment table as well as for those in wheelchairs. When performing a transverse plane seated technique, it is beneficial to obtain the compression phase of the technique (i.e., allow both hands to sink inwards), then take up the slack in an inferior direction, towards the client's pelvis.

Quick Questions

1. Is it necessary to look for red flare (a vasomotor response) during or after performing a transverse plane release technique?
2. What are the four main transverse planes in the human body?
3. What special issues must you address when performing the pelvic floor transverse plane release?
4. Can transverse plane release techniques be performed in any position other than lying on the treatment table?
5. For optimal results, what is the recommended amount of time for performing transverse plane release techniques?

Scar Tissue and Adhesion Management

MFR is used to treat restrictions and adhesions throughout the three-dimensional fascial network due to the dysfunction and pain caused by surgery or skin incision injury, or from overuse, misuse or abuse of the body. Because MFR treats body-wide dysfunction and pain, it is also effective and appropriate for the treatment of scar tissue and adhesion management.

Whilst surgery can cause a huge amount of scar tissue and adhesions, the invisible restrictions and adhesions throughout the body as a result of that incision injury or surgery can also cause ongoing system-wide dysfunction. An old hip injury, many years later, can cause restrictions and dysfunction in the ankle or shoulder due to compensatory patterns and fascial adhesions.

Scar tissue and adhesions from any injury creep throughout the system, sticking to pain-sensitive structures and causing tissues to adhere together. Often, nerves grow into the site of the adhesion or become enmeshed within the pull and drag of the adhesion, which then becomes painful.

The scar pictured in figure 10.1 shows how the tissue is different to the surrounding tissue. Skin scar tissue doesn't have hair follicles and is much paler than normal due to a reduced vascular supply.

This adherence creates further adhesions, compounding the dysfunction and creating a myriad of conditions.

Scar tissue can also cause more than just a physical effect on the body. Many people suffer from the emotional component of the original injury or surgery (i.e., the reason for the surgery or the cause of the injury), but the subsequent trauma, strain and stress as a result of the ongoing pain, discomfort and upset create a host of additional problems. Even the smallest scar, keyhole, injection site or incision can eventually create havoc within the delicate structures of the abdominal organs, nerves and blood vessels, which in turn can create so many of the symptoms seen in the treatment room.

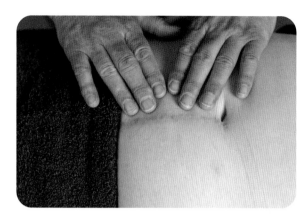

Figure 10.1 A mature scar.

All MFR techniques are safe to use on scar tissue and adhesions. However, specific techniques should be performed on the site of a scar at least six weeks after an injury or surgery. It is also appropriate to use MFR techniques prior to surgery. This potentially reduces adhesions already in that area but also has a calming influence on the client.

Many techniques are appropriate for scar tissue and adhesion management. The cross-hand release techniques are the most useful and can be performed above, below and across the scar site. Transverse plane techniques are beneficial for areas of tenderness and dense restriction, while specific scar techniques using the therapist's fingers apply a gentle, sustained pressure into the scar site itself. Other scar tissue techniques encourage gliding between layers, using a gentle lifting or tissue mobility approach.

As with all MFR, an integrative approach should be applied using different techniques to treat different tissue types and body parts.

Skin Rolling

As mentioned in chapter 4, skin rolling is an effective way to mobilise the tissue and to evaluate the skin and superficial fascia. It is also a great approach for the treatment of any adhesions, particularly abdominal ones, as a result of surgery or injury.

Skin rolling can be performed along either side of a scar and across it in many directions, and can also be done on the scar itself six weeks after an injury or surgery.

Skin rolling takes a bit of practice to get the rhythm right. It can be done in two general ways that are beneficial for the management of scars and adhesions: moving one hand and then the other, or moving both hands simultaneously.

Below is a review of skin rolling, which can also be found in chapter 4.

1. Begin by gently but securely grasping the tissue to one side of the scar between your finger pads and the thumbs of both hands.

2. Roll the tissue over your finger pads with your thumbs, one hand at a time or both together, walking your thumbs forwards and along the side of the scar.

3. Notice where the tissue feels stuck or is tender for your client. At these areas, wait and hold the tissue until you feel a sensation of softening, then begin to roll again.

4. Roll the skin slowly along the side of the scar in the same direction two or three times, then roll the skin in the other direction.

5. Repeat the process on the other side of the scar, then above and below the scar.

6. If the client is OK with you touching the scar, you can also roll the scar itself with one hand on one side on the scar and the other hand on the other side of the scar, with your hands as close together as possible so that you actually pick up the scar.

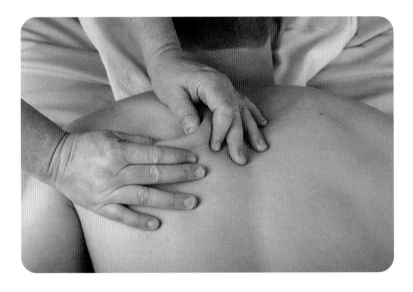

Skin Rolling the Abdominal Area

Skin rolling can also be used for anyone who has abdominal, digestive or bowel issues.

1. Skin roll the descending colon area first by starting inferior to the ribcage on the left hand-side of the abdomen and skin rolling down toward the pelvis.

2. Do this two or three times.

3. Next, skin roll the transverse colon, which is the area inferior to the ribcage across the upper abdomen. Skin roll from the right- to the left-hand side and continue down the descending colon.

4. Do this two or three times.

5. Finally, skin roll the ascending colon area superior to the pelvis on the right to the same side and continue across the transverse colon and down the descending colon.

6. Do this two or three times, effectively treating the descending colon the most.

This means that you are treating the descending colon first, followed by the transverse and then the ascending so that you are assisting any peristalsis of the colon towards the sigmoid colon and rectum on the left side of the body.

For smaller scars and keyhole surgery scars, you can skin roll right over the scar itself in multiple directions.

For burn scars and larger scars, take your time and skin roll from the periphery of the scar towards the middle of it. Sometimes, you need to treat larger scars over a number of sessions, and encourage the client to skin roll their own scars if they can reach them.

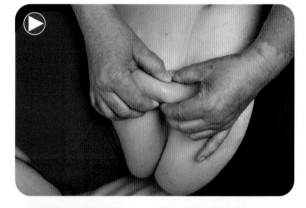

Some burn scars can feel thickened and difficult to skin roll, while others are thinner and more fragile. Take your time to assess how much of the tissue you can grasp gently between your fingers and thumbs before you roll the tissue so that the client doesn't feel any discomfort. Skin rolling in some areas can feel quite painful, so take care to skin roll very slowly and diligently.

Some areas of the skin will feel tighter and more adhered

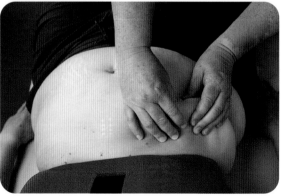

to the underlying tissues; this is normal in areas such as the feet, shoulder blades, backs and palms of the hands, and, for some people, the low back area. As a result, some areas of the body simply can't be skin rolled. Conversely, on some people, the low back area is very easy to skin roll, so it's not always about natural adherence but more that the tissue has become bound down to the tissue below.

Skin rolling is also an excellent technique for any scars and general tension on the face and neck. It is a great way to increase tissue movement and can be very relaxing to receive.

Position of Ease Techniques

Imagine one big restriction that is pulling all the tissue towards it. Distraction techniques traction, or pull, that tissue back out again (e.g., the leg or arm pull). Using a position of ease technique, you compress the tissue into the restriction to facilitate tissue change in the three-dimensional fascial matrix and then distract, or traction, the tissue back out again.

Position of ease techniques can be applied anywhere but are particularly good for scar tissue and adhesion management. These techniques are combined with either lifting the scar to tissue tension or leaning into the scar (e.g., compressing the tissues) to tissue tension.

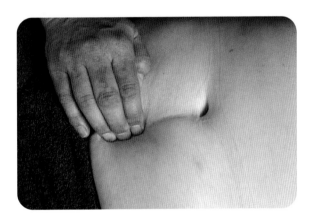

TIP Position of ease techniques rely on good kinaesthetic awareness because they are often very subtle. Take your time with these techniques to feel for tissue abnormality, and follow the path of least resistance.

Scar Lifting

Often, manual therapy techniques involve leaning into the tissue. Since scars tend to adhere layers of tissue together, it makes sense to separate these areas by lifting the tissue.

Like skin rolling, this is a simple but very effective technique. It is especially good for the abdominal area and as a mobilisation technique for scars on tendons such as the Achilles tendon.

Care should be taken to make sure that a scar is at least six weeks old before performing techniques directly on it.

Some small scars, where the tissue is reasonably thin, will only need one hand to perform this technique. Other scars will need both of your hands to support the tissue.

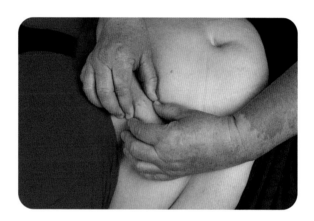

Keyhole and Small Scars

1. Gently grasp the scar with your fingers and thumb of one hand, as close to the scar site as you can.

2. Slowly and gently lift the tissue until you feel the tensional barrier of tissue resistance. Hold and wait at this barrier.

3. You may feel as if this barrier slowly melts and softens. Lift again to the tensional barrier of tissue resistance; hold and wait at this second barrier.

4. Maintaining this tissue resistance barrier, motion test the tissue in 12 o'clock, 3 o'clock, 6 o'clock and 9 o'clock positions to feel for the position of ease. A position of ease is a positional direction that the tissue favours and where you feel that the tissue moves towards with less resistance.

5. With the tissue lifted to the tensional barrier, and without letting the tissue drop down again, move the tissue gently away from you to the 12 o'clock position.

6. Remember what that sensation felt like, then return the tissue to the starting position.

7. Maintaining the tissue lift, gently take the tissue to the 3 o'clock position. Notice the feeling of tissue movement, then return it to the starting position.

8. Repeat the process to both the 6 o'clock and 9 o'clock positions.

9. Compare the four positions and determine to which position the tissue offered the least resistance.

10. The position that offered the least resistance is the one with which you start.

11. With the tissue lifted to tissue tension, move the tissue to its position of ease, and wait until you feel a subtle softening of the tissue. Move the tissue a little farther into its position of ease, waiting until you feel the second barrier melt and soften.

12. Add a second position of ease, that perpendicular to the initial position.

13. If your first position of ease was 12 o'clock, stay at 12 o'clock and motion test at 3 o'clock and 9 o'clock.

14. If your first position of ease was 3 o'clock, you are now going to motion test at 12 o'clock and 6 o'clock from that first position of ease.

15. If your first position of ease was 6 o'clock, you are now going to test for a position of ease at 3 o'clock and 9 o'clock from that first position of ease.

16. If your first position of ease was 9 o'clock, you are now going to test for a position of ease at 12 o'clock and 6 o'clock from that first position of ease.

17. This means that you have lifted the tissue to tissue tension, moved the tissue into a position of ease and then moved into a second position of ease perpendicular to the first.

18. This technique offers good results for scar tissue anywhere on the body and should take approximately three to five minutes to perform.

19. Dialogue with the client about any effects of and responses to the treatment.

If you are finding this difficult with your hands, the alternative is to use a small suction cup. Glass, plastic, silicone and rubber all work well. Simply place the cup onto the skin, create some suction and lift the tissue to tension in the same way as you would have done with your fingers and thumbs. Perform the technique in exactly the same manner as detailed above.

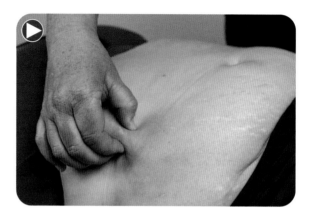

Long Scars

You can treat longer scars in exactly the same way as you would keyhole and smaller scars. This time you need both hands.

1. Gently lift the tissue, grasping the scar along its length in a pincer or key grip with your fingers on one side of the scar and your thumbs on the other side as close as possible to the scar site.

2. Slowly and gently lift the tissue until you feel the tensional barrier of tissue resistance. Hold and wait at this barrier.

3. You may feel as if this barrier slowly melts and softens. Lift again to the tensional barrier of tissue resistance. Hold and wait at this second barrier.

4. Maintaining this tissue resistance barrier, motion test the tissue in the 12 o'clock, 3 o'clock, 6 o'clock and 9 o'clock positions to feel for the position of ease. A position of ease is a positional direction that the tissue favours and where you feel the tissue moves towards with less resistance.

5. With the tissue lifted to the tensional barrier, and without letting the tissue drop down again, move the tissue gently away from you to the 12 o'clock position.

6. Remember what that sensation felt like, then return the tissue to the starting position.

7. Maintaining the tissue lift, now gently take the tissue to your 3 o'clock position. Notice the feeling of tissue movement, then return it to the starting position.

8. Repeat the process for both the 6 o'clock and 9 o'clock positions.

9. Compare the four positions and determine to which position the tissue offered the least resistance.

10. The position that offered the least resistance is the one with which you start.

11. With the tissue lifted to tissue tension, move the tissue to its position of ease, and wait until you feel a subtle softening of the tissue. Then move the tissue a little farther into its position of ease, waiting until you feel the second barrier melt and soften.

12. Add a second position of ease, that perpendicular to the initial position.

13. If your first position of ease was 12 o'clock, stay at 12 o'clock and motion test at 3 o'clock and 9 o'clock.

14. If your first position of ease was 3 o'clock, you are now going to motion test 12 o'clock and 6 o'clock from that first position of ease.

15. If your first position of ease was 6 o'clock, you are now going to test at 3 o'clock and 9 o'clock from that first position of ease.

16. If your first position of ease was 9 o'clock, you are now going to test at 12 o'clock and 6 o'clock from that first position of ease.

17. This means that you have lifted the tissue to tissue tension, moved the tissue into a position of ease and then moved into a second position of ease perpendicular to the first.

18. This technique should take you approximately three to five minutes to perform.

19. Dialogue with the client about any effects of and responses to the treatment.

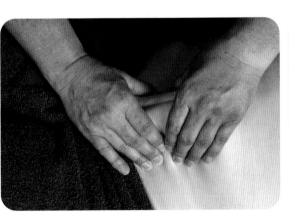
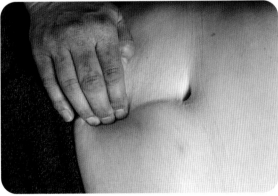

Compression Techniques for the Sternum

This technique is especially beneficial for clients with sternal scars from upper chest surgery, such as cardiac surgery. What is slightly different with this technique to the position of ease techniques is that you carry out the technique using the initial position of ease and then repeat the technique using the position of restriction.

1. Have the client lie supine on the treatment table.
2. Stand at the side of the treatment table.
3. Facing the client, place your hands one on of top of the other, skin on skin, onto the middle of the sternum.
4. Allow your hands to sink inwards to the tissue depth barrier, and apply a gentle pressure towards the client's head, noticing how much resistance is offered.
5. Slowly disengage your hands from the tissue, and move to stand at the top of the treatment table.
6. Place both your hands, one on top of the other, again on the client's sternum, and allow them to sink inwards to the tissue depth barrier.
7. Whilst maintaining an inward pressure, gently lean your pressure towards the client's feet, noticing how much resistance is offered.
8. Determine which direction offers a greater range of movement. This is the position of ease and the position in which to start the technique.
9. Re-place your hands on the client's sternum with your fingers pointing towards the position of ease, and allow them to sink inwards to the tissue depth barrier.
10. Whilst maintaining the inward pressure, at the same time gently direct your pressure towards the position of ease, waiting until you feel the tissue soften and yield, then slowly take up the slack and lean a little further towards the position of ease.

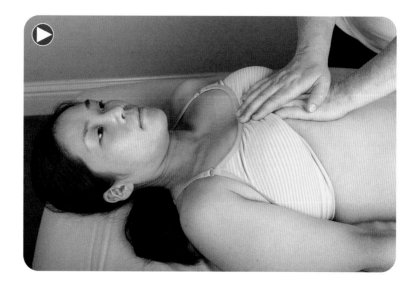

11. Remember not to force the barriers of tissue resistance or to slip over the skin.
12. Slowly remove your hands.
13. Repeat the technique, but this time start in the position of initial restriction.
14. Place your hands on the client's sternum with your fingers pointing towards the direction that offered the most resistance from your initial assessment, and allow them to sink inwards to the tissue depth barrier.
15. Whilst maintaining the inward pressure, at the same time gently direct your pressure towards the position of initial restriction, waiting until you feel the tissue soften and yield, then slowly take up the slack and lean a little further towards the position of initial restriction.
16. Wait approximately three to five minutes per direction for the tissue to change and soften.
17. Dialogue with the client about any effects of and responses to the treatment.

Compression Techniques for the Abdomen

The same technique for the sternum can be applied on the abdomen directly over a scar or on either side of it using your whole hand. Often, despite the injury or surgery being years old, clients still experience general tenderness and even bloating possibly due to internal adhesions. On the abdomen, you can add an additional position of ease.

1. Have the client lie supine on the treatment table.
2. Stand at the side of the treatment table.
3. Facing the client, place your hands one of top of the other, skin on skin, onto the abdominal scar.
4. Allow your hands to sink inwards to the tissue depth barrier, and apply gentle pressure towards the client's head, noticing how much resistance is offered.
5. Slowly disengage your hands from the tissue, and move to stand at the top of the treatment table.
6. Place both your hands, one on top of the other, again on the client's abdomen, and allow them to sink inwards to the tissue depth barrier.
7. Whilst maintaining an inward pressure, gently lean your pressure towards the client's feet, noticing how much resistance is offered.
8. Determine which direction offers a greater range of movement. This is the position of ease and the position in which to start the technique.
9. Re-place your hands on the client's abdomen with your fingers pointing towards the position of ease, and allow them to sink inwards to the tissue depth barrier.
10. Whilst maintaining the inward pressure, at the same time gently direct your pressure towards the position of ease, waiting until you feel the tissue soften

and yield, then slowly take up the slack and lean a little further towards the position of ease.

11. Remember not to force the barriers of tissue resistance or to slip over the skin.

12. Maintaining your depth and first position of ease, rotate or twist your hand slowly to your right, then allow your hand to come back to the starting point.

13. Rotate or twist your hand to your left, and determine which position offered the least resistance; this is the second position of ease.

14. Maintain your first position of ease and then add your second position of ease on top, holding your pressure gently at both tissue barriers.

15. You have now stacked two positions of ease: the depth barrier with a superior or inferior direction plus a twist, or rotation to the right or the left.

16. As you feel the tissue soften and yield, you may find that you can rotate or twist a little more to the next barrier or move more superiorly or inferiorly depending on your position of ease.

17. Once you have spent approximately three to five minutes with the tissue, starting from the inferior or superior first position of ease, go back and perform the technique again from the position that offered the most resistance. In other words, if the first position of ease was inferior, this time take the tissue superior and wait for it to soften.

18. Then, test for the position of ease with rotation; you will still move into the position of ease despite using the position of restriction with your previous hand placement.

19. Wait approximately three to five minutes with these last two stacked positions following any tissue changes offered.

20. Slowly disengage from the tissue.

21. Dialogue with the client about any effects of and responses to the treatment.

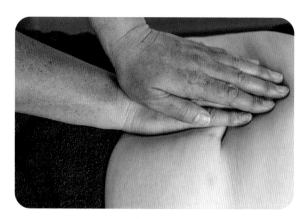

TIP Treating the abdomen can provide good outcomes, not just from abdominal surgery but also for hip and low back pain.

Treating the scar itself can be done with care and only after at least approximately six weeks after an injury or surgery. Some scars look like they are being sucked inwards, while others, such as a keloid scar, look like they pucker out. If you think of the way the tissue is being pulled or pushed, this is its position of ease. Therefore, position of ease techniques are applicable.

Option 1

1. Notice whether the visible scar is being sucked into the tissue or is lumpy or puckered.
2. The position of ease technique applies traction to a lumpy or puckered scar and compression to a scar that is sucked inwards.
3. If the tissue is being sucked in, use your fingers to engage the tissue and gently apply an inward pressure to the tissue resistance and depth barrier, following tissue changes three-dimensionally.
4. If the tissue is puckered or lumpy, gently take hold of the tissue and draw it towards you to the tissue resistance, following tissue changes in any direction.

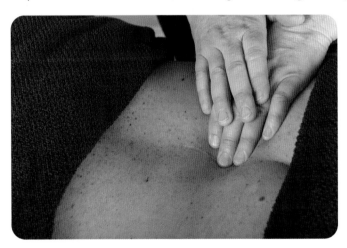

Option 2

1. Assess the scar by palpating along its length and obtaining feedback from the client as to which area is the most tender.
2. Begin the technique in the most tender area, sinking into the tissue resistance and depth barrier. Wait for the tissue to change three-dimensionally.
3. Reassess the scar and go to the next most tender area. Sink into the tissue, and wait for the tissue to change in any direction.
4. Continue until you have treated the entire scar.

Option 3

1. Assess the scar by palpating along its length and obtaining client feedback as to which area is the most tender.

2. Begin the technique in the most tender area, sinking your fingers into the tissue and applying pressure towards the 12 o'clock position, then 3 o'clock, 6 o'clock, and 9 o'clock. Obtain client feedback as to which direction is the most tender.

3. Starting in the direction which feels the most tender, lean inwards to the tissue depth barrier of resistance, and wait for the tissue to change and soften. Repeat the assessment process to find the next most tender area, again waiting patiently for tissue change.

4. Repeat in all directions until a significant reduction in discomfort occurs.

5. Finish with a cross-hand release technique.

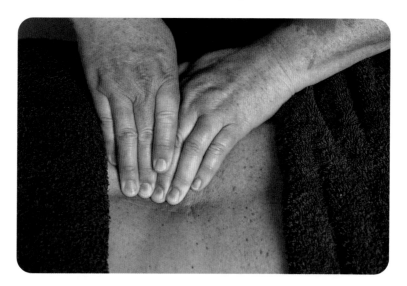

CLIENT TALK

Direct scar tissue work, although beneficial, can be quite painful and will elicit a burning sensation as the tissue changes. In many cases emotion can occur and should be encouraged as part of the process. MFR is an excellent therapy for treating scar tissue and adhesions, providing excellent results and relief for those in pain.

Closing Remarks

Treating clients who have scarring as a result of injury or surgery can be beneficial for the client and rewarding for the therapist.

Like all MFR, scar tissue treatments should be slow and diligent. Treating the body with MFR provides a whole-body approach. This means that we treat the entire person, not the condition or symptom. Resolving whole-body dysfunction and pain includes treating any scars regardless of their cause. Scars can affect existing body trauma and can sometimes be the cause of system-wide dysfunction. During the initial consultation, make sure you ask about any surgeries or injuries that have resulted in the formation of a scar.

Quick Questions

1. What's the minimum number of weeks to wait before directly treating a scar?
2. Which technique is an effective way to mobilise the tissue?
3. Is skin rolling good for treating abdominal adhesions that may have developed from abdominal surgery or injury?
4. Do position of ease techniques compress the tissue back towards the restriction?
5. What type of scar looks like it is puckered out from the skin?

Myofascial Mobilisations

Myofascial mobilisations, also known as soft tissue release (STR), pin and stretch, direct MFR and lever techniques, play another vital role in the integrated approach to MFR. Most myofascial mobilisations are applied in a longitudinal manner taking advantage of muscle lengthening adding either an active or passive muscle action over the joint. Alternatively, some are applied in a transverse manner, slowly separating and spreading the tissues either with or without movement of the joint.

In chapters 1 and 5, I discussed the differences between what some call the indirect and the direct approaches to MFR. The direct approach is another label for myofascial mobilisations and STR. Unfortunately, the label of 'direct' isn't descriptive of the techniques. Despite these ambiguous terms, the techniques are equally valuable.

CLIENT TALK

The myofascial mobilisations in this book are techniques that I have used for almost two decades in my own MFR practice and in MFR workshops. They are very effective for most but not all clients. Take your time applying them and always get client feedback. It's a good idea to combine myofascial mobilisations with the sustained approach to MFR so that you can offer the right treatment for every person.

Many myofascial mobilisations use a pin, hold or tissue lock with one hand or elbow and then add a stretch into the tissue, which can be either active or passive (see figure 11.1). From a functional point of view, adding movement to your treatment approach provides the client with proprioceptive feedback, enhancing motor control as well as providing an assessment of your treatment.

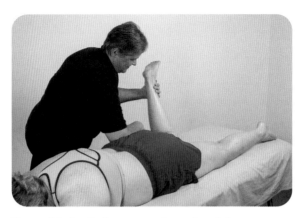

Figure 11.1 Piriformis myofascial mobilisation technique.

The fascial system plays a valuable role in both supporting and controlling active movement. According to the traditional biomechanical model, muscles move joints. However, musculoskeletal action is fully supported by the three-dimensional fascial system surrounding, encapsulating and permeating muscle. Fascia supports muscle action by helping the muscle to shorten by creating a radial stress around it and pulling it wider, thus shortening it.

This chapter discusses multi-directional techniques. Considering that the fascial system is a body-wide, three-dimensional matrix, assists muscle function and effectively widens the muscle, the best results will be obtained from multi-dimensional and multi-directional techniques, not simply longitudinal or transverse techniques.

None of these techniques use massage oil or lotion; this is not massage, which has more of a tendency to glide over the skin. The aim is to move very slowly and diligently through the tissue as you sense the tissue yielding to your pressure. The aim is to tune into your kinaesthetic awareness, feel the tissue quality below the skin and treat it effectively. When you feel you need to push or force to make any movement through the tissue, you need to wait at that tissue resistance, just as in the other MFR techniques earlier in the book. Only when the tissue yields to your pressure can you move a little farther through the tissues. The length of time this yielding takes can be very different from the right to the left sides of the body, let alone from person to person. This is what makes the integrated approach to MFR unique: you look, feel and treat individual areas of tension exclusive to that person.

The pressure used in myofascial mobilisations is not anywhere near as much as some therapists think. However, it is firmer than the pressure used for a cross-hand release or a transverse plane release technique described earlier in this book. Many of these techniques begin with what we call a broad stroke using the side of your elbow (not the point), a loose fist or the heel of your hand. These techniques are applied with your body weight so that you lean forward and down into the tissues, gently easing a gradual pressure into them. It is important not to push with your strength because this can be quite unpleasant for the client.

One important factor is the height of the treatment table when you apply these techniques. If your table is too high, you will just use the strength from your shoulder, upper arms and back, which eventually will become uncomfortable for you.

Once you have completed some broad strokes in slightly different directions to provide as much of a three-dimensional approach as you can, you can then become more specific, using thumbs, knuckles and fingers. However, note that using your fingers, thumbs and knuckles on a regular basis is not an ideal scenario for bodyworkers looking to maintain longevity in their careers. Using your digits must be done with care and with a slow, diligent application that does not force either your body or the client's tissue.

Applying Myofascial Mobilisation

These are the specific areas of the arms and hands that you use when applying myofascial mobilisations.

Elbow

This is the proximal third of the elbow, the area below the point of your elbow, called the olecranon. It is the area that consists of up to one third of the flexor compartment of your arm from the olecranon towards your wrist.

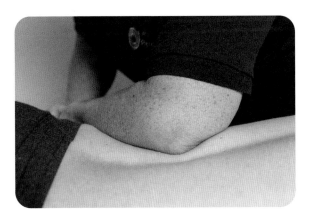

Olecranon

This is the point of your elbow.

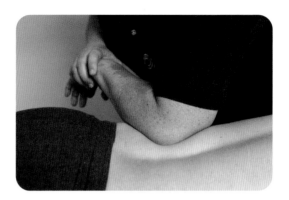

Side of Hand

This is the ulnar pinkie finger side of your hand.

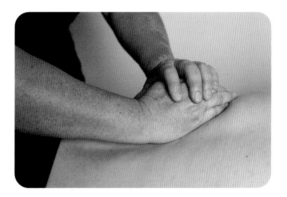

Heel of Hand

This is the area of your hand that is just above your wrist.

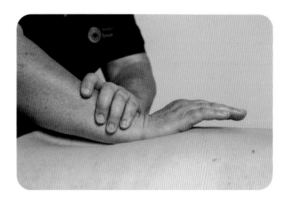

Loose Fist

Your hand should always stay relaxed, with the fingers loosely folded into the palm of the hand. Avoid clenching your fist, because that will be uncomfortable for you and even more so for the client. The part of your hand that makes contact with the client is the back of the fingers, called the proximal phalanges.

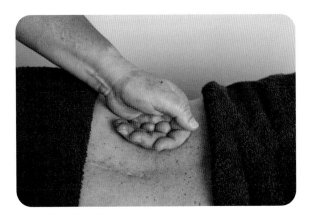

Supported Single Index Finger Knuckle

Any technique that uses your knuckles is not good for your fingers and feels uncomfortable for the client. However, using a supported single knuckle, usually your index finger, can be very effective *(a-b)*. Stack the joints of the finger below your wrist and elbow so that a directional pressure is applied from your shoulder instead of just using your knuckle.

Curl your index finger towards the palm of your hand and support it with your thumb and second finger like a brace on either side to protect it.

You can also support it with your other hand *(c)*.

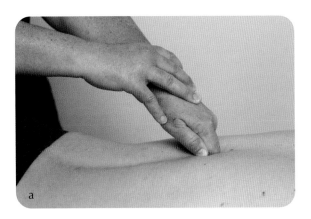

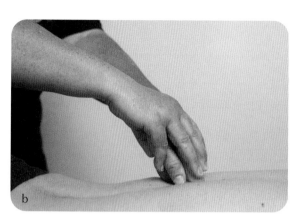
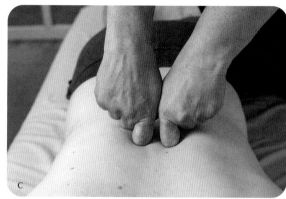

Curled Fingers

You will use your fingers for one technique. Close, or pack, the fingers close together so that they support each other.

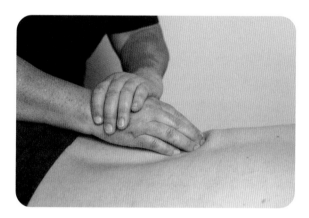

CLIENT TALK

When you apply myofascial mobilisation techniques, you have to choose the right tool—that is, the right part of your arm or hand—to perform the technique appropriately, obtain the best results and not injure yourself.

Ankle Retinacula

We are going to start with a very simple but valuable technique for the ankle. Foot and ankle stability is the foundation of the whole body.

The retinacula is a broad band of deep fascia that sits just at the top, or dorsum, of the foot. It is highly proprioceptive and holds the muscular tendons in place.

1. Have the client lie supine on the treatment table so that the ankles are slightly over the edge of the treatment table, allowing movement of the foot into dorsiflexion and plantar flexion.

2. Stand at the foot of the treatment table.

3. Ask the client to dorsiflex the foot and ankle you are going to treat so that the toes are pointing to the ceiling.

4. Using the proximal phalanges of your loose fists, place both your hands over the retinacula at the top of the foot close to the ankle.

5. Wait until you feel that your hands have contoured the ankle as much as possible, then ask the client to slowly point the toes into plantarflexion while you hold your position with your fists.

6. Once the client has plantarflexed as far as possible, release your pressure and ask the client to bring the toes back to the starting position.

7. Repeat the same process twice.

8. Ask the client to return the foot back to the starting position and re-place your hands. This time, as the client slowly plantarflexes, allow your hands to glide slowly towards either side of the ankle. Your movement won't be very far, but it will create a shearing effect on the tissues in a three-dimensional manner.

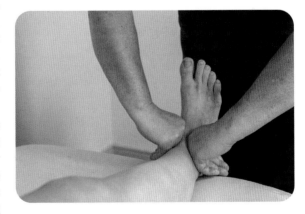

9. Once the client has plantarflexed as far as possible, release your pressure and ask the client to bring the toes back to the starting position.

10. Repeat the same process twice.

11. Apply the same technique to the other ankle and foot.

TIP If there is not enough space for both your hands on the retinacula, use just one hand at a time and perform the technique slowly, moving to one side of the ankle, then perform the technique again on the other side of the ankle.

Calf

This technique uses a transverse application, or a spreading, of the tissues.

1. Have the client lie prone on the treatment table with the ankle over the end of the table. You will be treating one leg at a time.
2. Stand at the bottom of the treatment table.
3. Ask the client to point the toes so that the foot and ankle are in plantar flexion.
4. Using loose fists, place them side by side over the bulkiest part of the client's calf where the gastrocnemius and soleus muscles are so the backs of your hands are almost touching.
5. Wait until you feel that your hands have contoured the leg as much as possible, then ask the client to slowly dorsiflex the ankle while you hold your position with your fists.
6. Once the client has dorsiflexed as far as possible, release your pressure and ask the client to bring the toes back to the starting position.
7. Repeat the same process twice.
8. Ask the client to return the foot back to the starting position and re-place your hands. This time, as the client slowly dorsiflexes, allow your hands to glide slowly towards either side of the leg. Your movement won't be very far, but it will create a shearing effect on the tissues in a three-dimensional manner.
9. Once the client has dorsiflexed as far as possible, release your pressure and ask the client to bring the toes back to the starting position.
10. Repeat the same process twice.
11. Move your loose fists closer towards the client's ankle and repeat the steps above three times without your hands moving and three times with your hands moving.

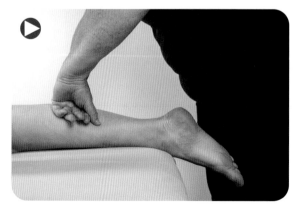 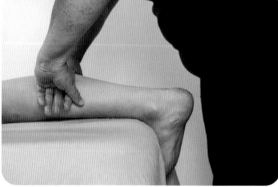

12. If there is space on their leg to do a third position closer towards their ankle, repeat the process one more time.

13. Repeat the same process on the opposite leg.

TIP If it feels better for your hands, you can use the heels of your hands instead to perform this technique in the same way.

Hamstring Muscle

This technique uses a transverse application, or a spreading, of the tissues.

1. Have the client lie prone on the treatment table.
2. Stand at the side of the treatment table next to the leg you will be working on.
3. Ask the client to bend the knee of the leg being treated to 90 degrees with the foot facing the ceiling.
4. You may need to ask the client to place the other leg into slight abduction, moving it away from the leg you are treating so there is space for your hands.
5. Place the heels of both your hands side by side over the client's hamstring muscle, just below the ischial tuberosity, so that the heels of your hands are almost touching.
6. Wait until you feel that your hands have contoured the leg as much as possible, then ask the client to slowly extend the knee to place the leg onto the treatment table while you hold your position with your hands.
7. Once the client has extended the leg, release your pressure and ask the client to bring the leg back to the starting position.
8. Repeat the same process twice.
9. Ask the client to return the leg back to the starting position and re-place your hands. This time, as the client slowly extends the leg, allow your hands to glide slowly towards either side of the leg. Your movement won't be very far, but it will create a shearing effect on the tissues in a three-dimensional manner.
10. Once the client has extended the leg, release your pressure and ask the client to bring the leg back to the starting position.
11. Repeat the same process twice.
12. Move your hands closer towards the client's knee and repeat the steps above three times without your hands moving and three times with your hands moving.
13. If there is space to do a third hand position closer again towards the client's knee, repeat the process one more time.
14. You also can do this technique using loose fists instead of the heels of your hands.

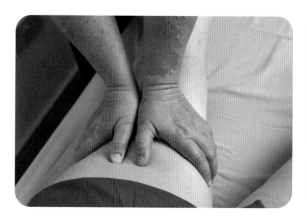 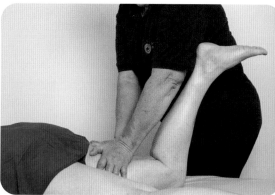

CLIENT TALK

Treating the hamstrings can be beneficial to everyone. We don't realise how much tension we hold here. Combine the myofascial mobilisation technique with a cross-hand release on the posterior thigh for maximum results.

TIP Some people have body hair on their legs, and it's important for you to apply these techniques slowly so that you don't pull at their body hair. If the client finds this painful, you might be using too much pressure. While these techniques are firmer than the cross-hand release and transverse plane techniques, they do not force or push at the tissue. You need to learn how to wait, follow and glide. Additionally, working through towels, sheets, or clothing can be done for modesty but makes it much harder on your hands and you lose your kinaesthetic awareness of what's happening under your hands. Try as much as possible to treat on their skin.

Quadriceps

This technique uses both a transverse, or a spreading, application of the tissues and a longitudinal application.

1. Have your client sit self-supported on a chair or on the treatment table by placing the hands on the chair or treatment table beside the hips.
2. Stand at the side of the leg you are going to work on.
3. Have the client extend the leg.
4. Place your loose fists side by side just above the client's kneecap.
5. Wait until you feel that your hands have contoured the leg as much as possible, then ask the client to slowly flex the knee while you hold your position with your hands.
6. Once the client has flexed the knee as far as possible, release your pressure and ask the client to bring the leg back to the starting position.

7. Repeat the same process twice.

8. Ask the client to return the leg to the starting position and re-place your hands. This time, as the client slowly flexes the knee, allow your hands to glide slowly towards either side of the leg, taking care of the normally tender areas of the adductors and the iliotibial band; your movement won't be very far, but it will create a shearing effect on the tissues in a three-dimensional manner.

9. Once the client has extended the leg, release your pressure and ask the client to bring the leg back to the starting position.

10. Repeat the same process twice.

11. Move your hands closer towards the client's body and repeat the steps above three times without your hands moving and three times with your hands moving.

12. There will be space to do a third and maybe even a fourth hand position closer towards their body for you to repeat the process.

13. Once you have done three or four hand placements up the leg, ask the client to return the leg to the starting position.

14. This time place the side of your elbow, the proximal third of your lower arm, just above the client's kneecap, with your hand pointing away from the client.

15. Wait until you feel that the side of your arm has contoured the leg as much as possible, then ask the client to flex their knee slowly while you slowly glide your arm up towards the client's body so that the speed of the knee flexion meets the speed of your arm moving slowly and diligently up the leg.

16. Slow knee flexion will give you the best results and will also be within the client's tolerance levels, so give the client clear direction on the speed they should use.

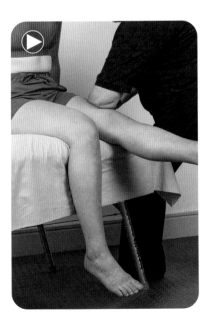
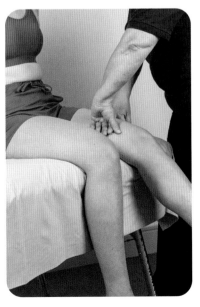

17. Once the client has flexed the knee as far as possible, release your pressure and ask the client to bring the leg back to the starting position.

18. Repeat the same process twice.

19. Repeat the process on the opposite leg.

TIP As in the hamstring technique, some clients have body hair on their upper legs. Take time to sink into the tissue so that you don't pull their hair.

CLIENT TALK

We usually think of treating legs for clients who are sporty. However, because the fascial compartments of the leg travel into the foot, treating legs can benefit anyone suffering from foot problems such as plantar fasciitis. Take your time and be diligent with the front and back of the legs, and complete the session with a longitudinal pull.

Seated Lateral Neck and Shoulder

This is a favourite technique of mine and one I learned on my own in MFR training at massage school. It's the technique that every student loves to receive and also the one from which clients derive so much benefit.

1. Have the client sit with a supported back without slouching. Use a pillow at the back if necessary.

2. Stand to the side of and slightly behind the client.

3. If you are standing on the right, place your right hand at the edge of the client's shoulder joint with your index finger on the clavicle and your thumb over the spine of the scapula. If you are standing on the left, use your left hand instead. This is your supporting hand, which also protects the bony landmarks.

4. With your opposite hand (working hand), contact the lateral neck with the proximal third of the flexor compartment of your forearm, with your hand facing over to their opposite shoulder away from the side you are treating.

5. Slowly and gently sink your body weight down to the floor with your working hand and engage the tissue.

6. Slowly begin to supinate your lower arm whilst maintaining your downward pressure.

7. Wait for the tissue to change and soften, then slowly sweep, or drag, the tissue in a controlled movement towards the acromioclavicular (AC) joint and your supporting hand.

8. The pace and pressure you give the client will feel firm but can often feel very pleasant and relieving.

9. Each fascial drag should take approximately 60 to 90 seconds to move from your starting point to reach the AC joint, or longer if the tissue is tight.

10. Repeat three or four times.
11. Next, ask the client to laterally flex the head slowly away from the side you are treating to increase the stretch.
12. Ask the client to bring the head and neck back to the starting point before removing your pressure.
13. You can also ask the client to do the same with head and neck rotation.
14. Repeat on the other side.

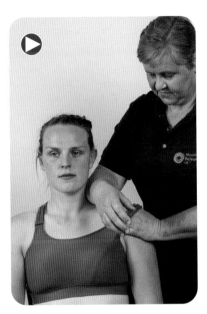 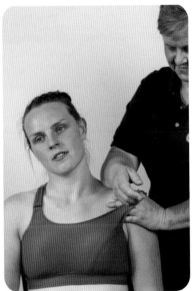

Seated Upper Trapezius

This is a transverse technique to spread the tissues.

1. Have the client sit with a supported back without slouching. Use a pillow at the back if necessary.
2. Stand to the side of and face behind the client.
3. Contact the lateral neck with the proximal third of the flexor compartment of your forearm so that your hand is facing behind the client.
4. Ask the client to extend the head and neck slightly to a comfortable position.
5. Lean slowly and gradually down onto the top of the client's shoulder.
6. Wait for the tissue to change and soften, then slowly drag the tissue down the upper back.
7. As you are slowly dragging down the upper back, ask the client to slowly drop the head forwards into flexion, tucking the chin as close to the chest as possible.

8. Continue to drag your arm slowly and in a controlled manner down the upper back between the scapula and the spine, waiting for the tissue to let you move. You will only need to move about 2 to 2.5 inches (5–6 cm) at the most.

9. Ask the client to lift the head to the starting position, then release your pressure.

10. Repeat the process three or four times at a very slightly different angle so that you are making a fan shape from the client's shoulder onto the upper back, taking care not to push or lean onto the scapula.

11. Repeat on the opposite shoulder.

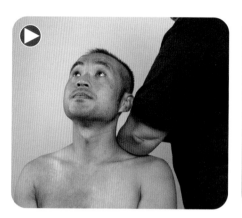 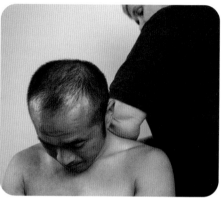

TIP As you slowly drag down the upper back, some people are so tight here that you can only move about 0.8 to 1.2 inches (2–3 cm). This area can be sensitive, and some will push their shoulders up to resist your pressure. This is an immediate clue to lighten your pressure and start slower, gradually leaning further into the tissue as it changes.

Erector Spinae Muscle

This technique uses a longitudinal application.

1. Have your client sit on a sturdy stool or on a chair with a flat base.

2. Ask the client to drop the arms down by the sides and place feet flat on the floor, shoulder-width apart. Ideally, the knees should be lower than the hips to allow the client to perform adequate hip flexion when bending over.

3. Stand behind the client so that you are in a lunge stance, and place the proximal third of your lower arm onto the erector spinae on either side of the spine at C7-T1 (over the upper trapezius if possible).

4. Lean into the client's body and wait for the tissue to yield.

5. Ask the client to drop chin to chest and slowly begin to roll forward, not flexing at the hips but flexing the spine, vertebra by vertebra. The client should keep the arms at the sides and create a counter pressure through the feet up the body to meet your pressure.

6. Slowly begin to drag your arms down the client's back, staying on the erector spinae muscles on either side of the spine.

7. Your inferior movement through the tissue is guided by the pace of the client's body as it flexes forward. You may need to be specific with your guidance on the speed of the movement.

8. If the client resists your pressure too much, you will feel the need to push back. Your pressure should be relatively firm feeling for tissue tension but not using force. You need to create a balance between the client's body and your elbows. Don't work too hard.

9. Make sure the client moves slowly as you slowly take up the slack feeling for the tissue yielding, allowing you to move inferiorly.

10. Take care as you reach the lumbar spine because these vertebrae are wider than those above. It can take approximately 60 to 90 seconds to compete one movement from the top to the bottom of the back. If you go too fast, you might apply more than the client can tolerate.

11. Once you have reached the last vertebra, remove your elbows and ask the client to roll slowly upwards, focusing on each vertebra at a time.

12. Repeat the same process twice with your elbows or loose fists.

13. Repeat the same process with the knuckle of your index fingers bilaterally applied to the lamina groove between the spinous process and the erector spinae muscle. Take care not to extend the knuckle at the metacarpal phalangeal joints; rather, curl all the finger joints.

14. For any further restrictions, focused release with your elbows or knuckles can be performed in the same manner as above. Additions might include active flexion and extension of the spine and active rotation to further the release.

15. Please take time with this technique. It should be done slowly and diligently.

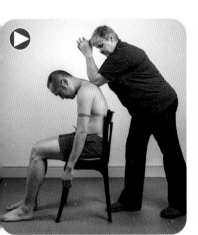
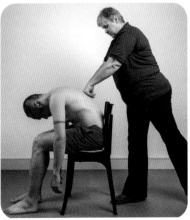
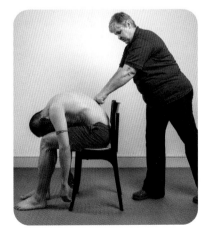

CLIENT TALK

This is an exceptionally good technique not just for treating the back, but for the legs, feet, and head and neck. Combine this technique with the seated upper trapezius technique, then finish with longitudinal arm pull with the client lying supine.

Pectoralis Muscle

This is a transverse technique.

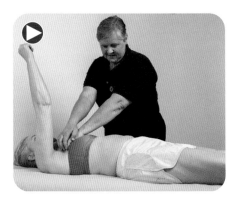

1. Have the client lie supine on the treatment table.

2. Stand on the opposite side of the treatment table to the side you are going to treat.

3. Reach across with both hands to contact the lateral edge of the pectoralis major muscle.

4. You can use one hand or place your hands one on top of the other.

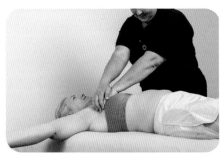

5. Female clients can also assist with this technique by placing their own hand on the opposite pectoralis major muscle, and then you place one of your hands on top.

6. Ask the client to place the arm into the air so that the hand and fingers point to the ceiling.

7. Gently and slowly lean backwards, slightly dragging the tissue towards you, then ask the client to slowly drop the arm out to the side as in horizontal extension or abduction of the shoulder joint; this will lengthen the tissue.

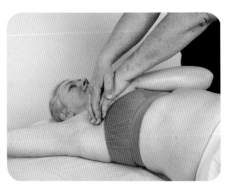

8. Once the client has reached as far as possible, slowly release your pressure.

9. Ask the client to return the arm to the starting position, and re-place your hands on the lateral border of the pectoralis muscle.

10. Slowly repeat the stretch another two times.

11. Ask the client to place the arm into the air so that the hand and fingers point to the ceiling.

12. Re-place your hands, but this time ask the client to take the arm out to the side but at a slightly higher angle towards the head.

13. Repeat at this angle two or three times.

14. Repeat this technique in three or four different angles of the arm in a fan shape; this will assist with tissue change and lengthening of the muscle.

15. Repeat on the other side.

Psoas and Iliacus

Please do not use this technique on someone who is pregnant or trying to become pregnant.

This is a longitudinal and a transverse technique.

1. Have your client lie supine on the treatment table.

2. Ask the client to bend the knee on the side you will be treating and rest it towards their other leg in adduction.

3. Palpate to find their anterior superior iliac spine (ASIS) and the iliac crest on this side.

4. Slide your fingers slowly and gently just inside the iliac crest adjacent to the ASIS to contact the iliacus muscle.

5. Wait for the tissue to change and yield, then slowly move your fingers medial and inferior until you feel you can't go any further without forcing the tissue.

6. Ask the client to slowly bring the knee to chest so you can feel the iliopsoas contracting under your finger as the hip flexes.

7. If you do not feel the contraction, lift your fingers slowly up and out of the tissue and replace them slightly more medially and inferiorly.

8. Wait for the tissue to yield, then ask the client to bring the knee to chest as you feel for the iliopsoas contracting.

9. You may need to use this assessment approach two or three times until you locate the iliopsoas muscle.

10. Once you have located the iliopsoas, gently and slowly apply posterior pressure into the muscle and wait for the tissue to yield.

11. Ask the client to flex the other knee, placing both heels close to the buttocks with knees bent and feet together on the treatment table.

12. Ask the client to perform five to six slow, repetitive anterior and posterior pelvic tilts.

13. You will feel the iliopsoas contract with this movement. Retain your pressure on the muscle during this movement.

14. Ask the client to slowly bring the knee to chest on the side you are treating so that you can feel the iliopsoas muscle contracting; this lets you know that your fingers are still in the right place. If you can't feel the iliopsoas contracting, re-place your fingers to locate it.

15. With the client's knees bent, ask them to slowly lift their buttocks to the ceiling, just lifting a few inches or centimetres off the treatment table, then slowly replace their buttocks on the treatment table.

16. Repeat this movement two to three times as you maintain your pressure on the iliopsoas muscle.

17. Ask the client to slowly bring the knee to their chest on the side you are treating so that you can feel the iliopsoas muscle contracting; this lets you know that your fingers are still in the right place. If you can't feel the iliopsoas contracting, re-place your fingers to locate it.

18. Next, ask the client to allow the leg you are not treating to extend flat onto the treatment table while the leg you are treating remains flexed at the knee.

19. With your fingers still on the iliopsoas muscle, ask the client to allow you to slowly lengthen this leg into an extended position.

20. Place your free hand onto the ankle and very slowly slide their foot down the treatment table. Don't lift the leg up; rather, guide their leg into a straightened position.

21. This will feel like a stretch with your fingers pinning, or locking, the iliopsoas muscle.

22. Once the leg is straight, lift your pressure off the iliopsoas slightly and place the client's leg back once again in a flexed position at the knee with their foot placed onto the treatment table as before.

23. Ask the client to slowly bring the knee to chest so that you can feel the iliopsoas muscle contracting; this lets you know that your fingers are still in the right place. If you can't feel the iliopsoas contracting, re-place your fingers to locate it.

24. Repeat the process of straightening the client's leg followed by flexing at the knee again two more times.

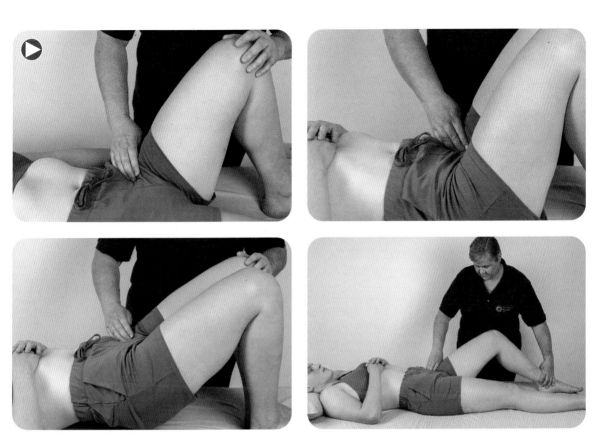

TIP Not all clients can tolerate the different components of this technique in one treatment session. The components can be broken down to only one or two of them in one session; they don't all have to be done in succession.

Treating the iliopsoas muscle has its critics. Some people suggest that iliopsoas cannot be accurately palpated through the overlying tissues while others suggest that the intestinal organs may be compromised. I was taught to treat iliopsoas at the level of the umbilicus. This is no longer taught in most manual therapy schools. I do believe that iliopsoas can be distinguished from other tissues by skilled hands, but I also suggest extreme caution and care performing this technique. Take your time to learn it and also take your time applying it with every client.

Piriformis

This is a transverse and longitudinal technique.

1. Have the client lie prone on the treatment table.
2. Contact the lateral edge of the piriformis. To find the piriformis, draw an imaginary line between the anterior superior iliac spine (ASIS) and the coccyx and another line between the posterior superior iliac spine (PSIS) and the most prominent point of the greater trochanter. Where these two lines cross is the belly of the piriformis.
3. Glide laterally from this point towards the greater trochanter so that you are lateral to the belly of the muscle and closer to its insertion at the greater trochanter.
4. Using the proximal third of your elbow, a loose fist or the heel of your hand, palpate to locate the piriformis and slowly sink down anteriorly into the tissue. Wait for the tissue to yield and soften.
5. Ask the client to flex the knee.
6. As you maintain your pressure, ask the client to slowly internally and externally rotate the upper leg at the hip in small movements about 8 to 10 times.
7. If the client begins to tire, you can take hold of the ankle and move the leg yourself in a passive action.
8. Next, with the client's leg flexed at the knee again, also place it into external rotation of the hip, which will shorten the piriformis.
9. Pin, or lock, the piriformis muscle with the proximal third of your elbow, a loose fist or heel of your hand and wait for the tissue to feel like it is softening.
10. Move the client's leg slowly into internal rotation of the hip to stretch the piriformis without removing your pressure.
11. Release your pressure slightly once you have moved the leg into internal rotation as far as it will go.

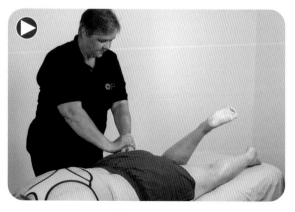
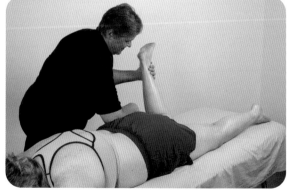

12. Position the client's leg back into external rotation and once again apply pressure to the piriformis muscle.

13. Without removing your pressure, move the leg slowly back into internal rotation of the hip.

14. Release your pressure and repeat another two to three times.

CLIENT TALK

The piriformis technique is a very valuable technique because so many clients have hip, low back and pelvic issues. Take care to complete a full consultation of the client's complaints of pain in this area and rule out sciatica using appropriate testing.

Gluteus Medius, Gluteus Minimus and Tensor Fascia Lata

This is a transverse technique.

1. Have the client lie on their side on the treatment table.

2. Palpate the client's hip to locate the tensor fascia lata (TFL) and the gluteus medius and minimus muscles. These muscles can be found by asking the client to abduct the leg up and off the treatment table.

3. Ask the client to bring both their legs towards their chest with slight hip flexion, so that they are comfortable and stable on the treatment table.

4. Using the proximal third of your lower arm, a loose fist or the heel of your hand, palpate to locate the TFL muscle and slowly apply pressure towards the floor (medial) into the tissue and wait for a sense of tissue change and softening.

5. While maintaining your pressure, ask the client to very slowly straighten the leg on the side being treated without lifting it towards the ceiling, then slowly replace it back on to the other leg.

6. Repeat this two or three times.

7. While maintaining your pressure, ask the client to straighten the leg as before and to slightly lift it towards the ceiling just a couple of inches or centimetres, then place it back down.

8. It is important to do this slowly and in a controlled manner to stop the client from rolling forwards.

9. Repeat this two or three times.

10. Slowly remove your pressure and locate the gluteus minimus and medius muscles slightly posterior and inferior to the placement of TFL.

11. Using the proximal third of your lower arm, a loose fist or the heel of your hand, slowly apply pressure towards the floor (medial) into the tissue and wait for a sense of tissue change and softening.

12. While maintaining your pressure, ask the client to very slowly straighten the leg on the side being treated without lifting it towards the ceiling, then slowly replace it back on to the other leg.

13. Repeat this two or three times.

14. While maintaining your pressure, ask the client to straighten the leg as before and to slightly lift it towards the ceiling a couple of inches or centimetres, then place it back down. It is important to do this slowly in a controlled manner so the client doesn't roll forwards.

15. Repeat this two or three times.

16. Slowly remove your pressure and move the proximal third of your lower arm, a loose fist or the heel of your hand slightly farther posterior on the client's hip and pelvis and also inferiorly to locate the gluteus medius muscle.

17. Using the proximal third of your lower arm, a loose fist or the heel of your hand, slowly apply pressure towards the floor (medial) into the tissue and wait for the tissue to change and soften.

18. While maintaining your pressure, ask the client to very slowly straighten the leg on the side being treated without lifting it towards the ceiling, then slowly replace it back on to the other leg.

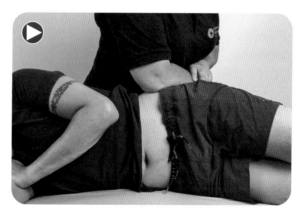

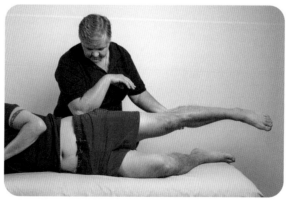

19. Repeat this two or three times.

20. Ask the client to straighten the leg as before and to slightly lift it towards the ceiling just a couple of inches or centimetres, then place it back down.

21. Repeat this two or three times.

TIP As with the iliopsoas technique, this technique can be completed in stages so that it is always done within client tolerance.

Closing Remarks

Myofascial mobilisations are a great addition to the MFR repertoire and are probably the most traditional style of MFR. The most important thing to remember with these techniques is that, like the sustained approach to MFR such as the cross-hand release technique, less is more. The fact that you are using an elbow, knuckle or fist doesn't mean that you push or force. It's actually the opposite. Taking more time and being very diligent and slow with these techniques provides valuable and effective results.

Quick Questions

1. What are three of the other names commonly used for myofascial mobilisations?
2. In which two main directions are myofascial mobilisations performed?
3. What are the proximal phalanges?
4. Which two muscles are we mainly treating when we treat the calf muscle?
5. Should you do the iliopsoas myofascial mobilisation technique on a person who is or is trying to become pregnant?

PART IV

MFR Programmes and Management

This final part of the book addresses combining the previously discussed techniques so that you can see how they can fit together as a treatment approach, helping you refine your skills. While MFR does not include protocols for specific groups of techniques, some techniques seem like they are a natural fit. Being able to move fluidly from one technique to the next offers confidence to the client and helps you build your technique repertoire.

Chapter 12 discusses how to combine techniques and gives you some ideas of which ones fit well together for you to practise. It also provides some additional information regarding the position of ease techniques used for scar tissue in chapter 10 so that you can see how to use this approach for tissue assessment. Chapter 13 offers information about individual and multi-therapist MFR treatment sessions as well as management of home care myofascial programmes, which clients (or you) can use between MFR treatment sessions.

Combined Techniques and Taking MFR Further

This chapter describes techniques you have seen before but offers additional information and variations on a theme to enhance your MFR skills. You have already practised some fundamental, easy-to-use and effective techniques. Now you will learn how to combine techniques including specific techniques to balance the physical structure of the body, improving both form and function.

Although I suggest certain technique combinations, continue to use your intuition and felt sense awareness and follow the needs of your client, never forcing the tissue barrier or slipping or gliding over the skin. Always perform any techniques for three to five minutes for optimal results.

Chapter 10 addressed position of ease techniques for treating scar tissue in more detail. Following is a simple assessment and two techniques for you to use on the tissue.

Tissue Motion Test

Before applying a position of ease technique, you need to motion test the tissue. As with all MFR techniques, remember to set your intention, connect with yourself and the client, tell the client what you are going to do and look for, and ask about any response to the treatment. Read through the technique so that you understand the application before performing it.

1. Have the client lie supine on the treatment table.
2. Perform the entire technique from the same side of the treatment table. Alternatively, you can position yourself so that your hands are always pushing away from you by performing one phase of the technique on one side of the table and the second phase from the opposite side.
3. Place your hands on the client's body, allowing them to soften into the tissue to the depth barrier in the same manner as in a cross-hand release technique.
4. Motion test the tissue by taking up the slack (taking the tissue with you and not gliding on the skin) in the direction the technique requires.
5. Keep your hands on the tissue and allow them to drift back to your starting point, then take up the slack in the opposite direction, again taking the tissue with you and not gliding on the skin. Determine which direction offered greater movement.
6. Always start the technique in the direction that offered the greater range, which will allow you to compress the tissues into the lesion rather than tractioning them back out.

Leg Roll Position of Ease

1. Have the client lie supine on the treatment table.
2. Stand at the side of the treatment table.
3. Place both of your hands side by side on the client's anterior thigh, allowing your hands to sink inwards to the tissue depth barrier in the same way as you do in the first part of the cross-hand release technique. Remember not to slip over the skin or force the barrier.
4. Maintaining that pressure, begin to medially rotate, or internally roll, the client's leg, making sure that the movement comes from the hip joint. Notice how far you can roll the leg inwards.
5. Keep your hands on the client's leg, and allow the leg to return to neutral.
6. Roll the leg externally or laterally rotate it, and again notice how far it moves.
7. Determine whether the leg rolls more easily medially or laterally.
8. Begin the technique in the direction you feel offers greater movement.

9. Standing so you can roll the leg away from you, re-place your hands on the client's anterior thigh, allowing your hands to sink inwards to the tissue depth barrier.

10. Take up the slack to the tissue resistance in your position of ease, waiting for the tissue to soften and yield both inwards and either laterally or medially.

11. Every time the tissues soften and yield, take the tissue a little further into its position of ease.

12. Dialogue with the client about any effects of and responses to the treatment.

13. Once you have gained a significant tissue change in the first phase of the technique, stand at the side of the treatment table so you can roll the client's leg away from you and use the same process in the direction that offered the least movement.

14. Wait approximately three to five minutes per side for the tissue to change.

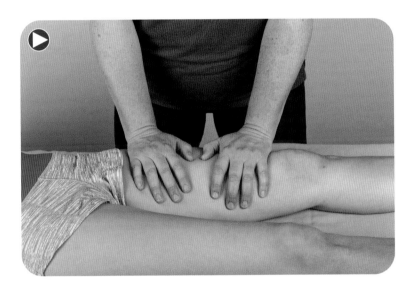

Seated Thoracolumbar Junction Position of Ease

1. Have the client sit tall, not slouching, at the end of the treatment table, with the feet supported if necessary.

2. Stand at the side of the treatment table.

3. Place one of your hands, skin on skin, at approximately T12, the thoracolumbar junction, and place your other hand, skin on skin, at the angle of the ribs at the end of the sternum. This is the same hand position as the respiratory diaphragm transverse release technique.

4. Allow both of your hands to sink into the client's tissue to the tissue depth barrier.

5. Begin to slowly rotate the thoracic cage away from you, making sure the client does not try to help you. Notice how much movement is offered.

6. Allow the ribcage to come back to neutral, then rotate it towards you. Notice how much movement is offered. Maintain the tissue depth barrier at all times.

7. Determine whether the ribcage moves more easily to the right or to the left.

8. Begin the technique in the direction you feel offers greater movement. Remember not to slip over the skin or force the barrier.

9. Perform this technique standing at the side of the treatment table so you can roll the ribcage away from you easily.

10. Re-place your hands on the client's ribcage, again allowing them to sink into the client's tissue to the tissue depth barrier.

11. Take up the slack in your position of ease to the point of tissue resistance, maintaining your tissue depth barrier. Wait for the tissue to feel like it softens and yields, then begin to rotate the ribcage away from you as the tissue continues to change.

12. Dialogue with the client about any effects of and responses to the treatment.

13. Once you have gained a significant tissue change in the first phase of the technique, slowly bring the client back to neutral, move to the opposite side of the treatment table and apply the same process in the direction that offered you the least movement. Keep rotating the ribcage away from you as the tissue softens and accommodates this movement until a significant softening of the tissue has occurred.

14. Wait approximately three to five minutes per side for the tissue to change.

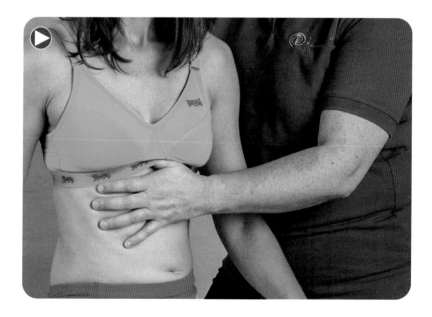

Lower Body Option 1

1. Have the client sit on a stool or chair, and perform a myofascial mobilisation for the erector spinae muscles, described in chapter 11.

2. Ask the client to lie supine on the treatment table and move the hip on the side to be treated to the edge of the treatment table and to hang the leg over the edge. The opposite knee and hip are bent to support the low back.

3. Stand at the side of the treatment table, and hook your lower leg around the client's lower leg.

4. Place your hands in the position of a cross-hand release of the anterior hip, and perform that technique slowly and gradually, sinking into the tissue as it softens and yields. Remember not to slip over the skin or force the barrier.

5. Dialogue with the client about any effects of and responses to the treatment.

6. Once you have gained a significant softening of the tissue, gently lift the client's leg back onto the treatment table, then take the leg through the leg pull technique described in chapter 7. You may need to have the client move back to the middle of the treatment table to perform the leg pull.

7. Ensure that you perform each technique for at least three to five minutes for optimal results.

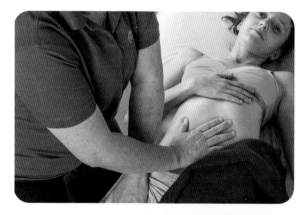

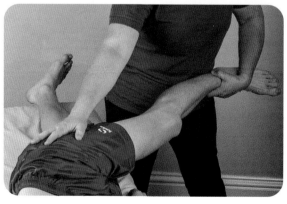

Upper Body Option 1

1. Have the client sit, and perform a myofascial mobilisation of the lateral neck and shoulder technique, described in chapter 11.

2. Have the client lie supine on the treatment table with the arm on the side you are working on externally rotated so that the palm is facing upwards. This arm should hang slightly over the edge of the treatment table.

3. Stand at the top of the treatment table.

4. Place your hands in the position of a cross-hand release of the anterior upper chest, and perform that technique, sinking into the tissue as it softens and yields. Remember not to slip over the skin or force the barrier.

5. Dialogue with the client about any effects of and responses to the treatment.

6. Once you have gained a significant tissue change, move to the side of the treatment table and perform an arm pull, following all the tissue changes as it softens and yields to your touch.

7. Ensure that you perform each technique for at least three to five minutes for optimal results.

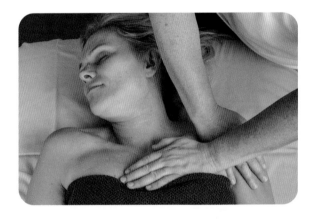

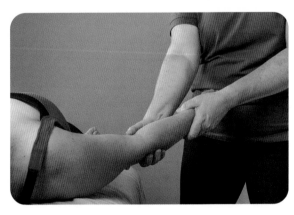

Lower Body Option 2

1. Have the client sit in a chair or on the treatment table, and on both legs perform a myofascial mobilisation of the quadriceps muscle, described in chapter 11.
2. Have the client lie prone on the treatment table, and on both legs perform a myofascial mobilisation of the calf muscle, described in chapter 11.
3. Have the client lie supine on the treatment table, and perform either a single or bilateral leg pull technique.

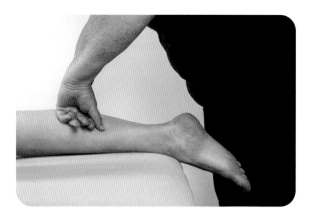

Lower Body Option 3

1. Have the client lie prone on the treatment table, and perform a myofascial mobilisation of the piriformis muscle, described in chapter 11.
2. On the same leg, perform a cross-hand release of the posterior thigh, described in chapter 6.
3. Perform a prone leg compression technique, described in chapter 8.
4. Dialogue with the client about any effects of and responses to the treatment.
5. Ensure that you perform each technique for at least three to five minutes for optimal results.

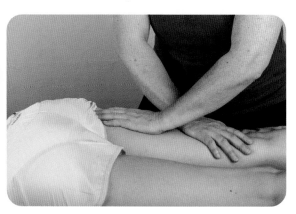
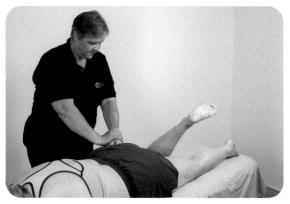

Lower Body Option 4

1. Have the client lie supine on the treatment table, and begin to skin roll the abdominal area, starting with the descending colon, followed by the transverse colon and the ascending colon, as described in chapter 10.

2. Perform the transverse plane release of the respiratory diaphragm technique described in chapter 9.

3. Perform a supine bilateral leg pull, described in chapter 7.

4. Dialogue with the client about any effects of and responses to the treatment.

5. Ensure that you perform each technique for at least three to five minutes for optimal results

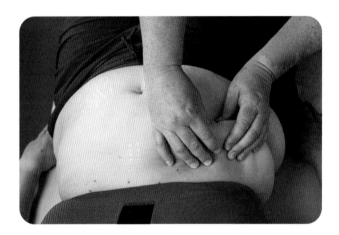

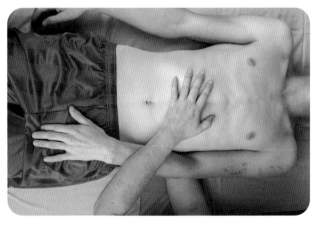

Upper Body Option 2

1. Have the client sit on a stool or chair and perform a myofascial mobilisation for the erector spinae muscles and a lateral neck and shoulder technique, described in chapter 11.

2. Perform a cross-hand release of the upper chest (pectoralis area) either doing both sides together or one side at a time, described in chapter 6.

3. Perform a supine bilateral arm pull, described in chapter 7.

4. Dialogue with the client about any effects of and responses to the treatment.

5. Ensure that you perform each technique for at least three to five minutes for optimal results

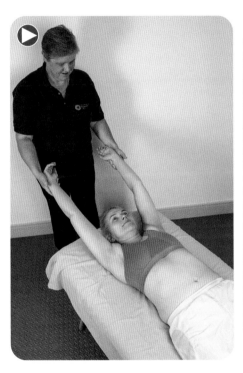
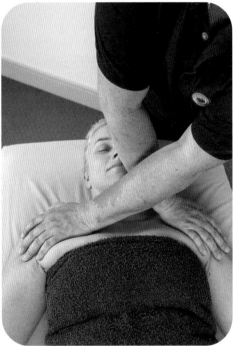

Closing Remarks

You now have excellent techniques to practise that will help you expand your knowledge and experience of working with the entire fascial matrix. As your skills develop, you will begin to realise that where your hands are, how you position the client and how you perform the technique are not the most important aspects of any treatment. More important are where you feel your hands should be placed, what you notice happening in response to the treatment, what you do with that response and how you work with the client in a unique way. This results in a holistic approach to health. An experienced MFR therapist said to me, 'Allow the work to be organic'.

Every technique can be performed in so many ways depending on you and your client. This is why MFR is considered an art form. You can learn the basics and the theory and understand how to apply the techniques, but you will only make it your own with practice.

Every technique can be integrated with others. You may prefer some techniques over others, and some you may change to suit your needs and your clients' requirements. Experiment with the techniques offered here and blend them, but most of all, listen to what your hands are telling you and follow where they are being led.

Receiving MFR treatments yourself and attending hands-on MFR workshops will enhance everything you are learning in this book.

Quick Questions

1. Which techniques can you combine?
2. In which position do you start the position of ease myofascial techniques?
3. Despite skin rolling being part of an assessment for restrictions, can it be integrated as a technique with all other MFR techniques?
4. How can you enhance your experience of MFR?
5. What is the optimum time length for performing the indirect style of MFR?

MFR Treatment Approaches

All treatment approaches, whether individual, intensive or multi-therapist, follow the same basic format and are influenced by the experience and ability of the therapist(s). Receiving any kind of therapy will be determined by a number of factors including the fact that even though the client may be in pain, the result of any treatment will depend on the client's ability to attend enough sessions to experience the desired results.

If you take the time to help clients understand the MFR approach, the basic role of fascia in the body and why the structure must be balanced from top to toe to eliminate the pain, they will be more likely to embrace the approach and work with you to facilitate the treatment. Having articles, books, brochures and flyers about MFR available for clients to take home, buy or borrow is an excellent way to help them understand the MFR approach.

CLIENT TALK

Clients often ask, 'How long will it take?' and 'How many sessions will I need?' The truth is that you do not know how any client is going to respond until you have worked together for a few sessions. It would be unfair and unrealistic to tell a client that two sessions will fix the issue, yet you need to make some reference to a positive progression. You don't want clients in chronic pain to believe that they will never get better; however, you do want to be as realistic as possible and help them understand that you have to work together to get them where they want to go.

Individual Treatment Approaches

In individual treatment approaches, one therapist works with one client, and the client receives one session at a time, perhaps once a week or once a month. If a few therapists share a clinic, the client may see different therapists during the course of treatment; however, individual treatment generally consists of one-on-one hands-on treatments that are usually an hour long.

MFR, unlike other therapies, does not have a set number of treatment sessions. Discomfort can resolve after three or four sessions for some clients; other clients may need more. Every client is unique, but generally, how long the person has had discomfort and dysfunction determines the length of time required to undo emotional bracing patterns and the habitual holding patterns built up over time to compensate for the original injury.

Ideally, treatment sessions should be no less than an hour in length, although this may not be possible in some clinics or hospitals. In such cases the therapist has to maximise the time available. Some clients, because of work and family commitments and financial constraints, are not able to attend therapy on a regular basis. Such clients need to understand that you will always do your best and that progress will happen, albeit more slowly than it would with more regular treatments. Encourage clients to commit to at least three sessions as close together as possible so they will have regular therapy for at least a while.

Individual treatment sessions are beneficial to clients who are physically not well enough to attend more than one hour at a time. If you can manage to give these clients at least some MFR, they may start attending more regularly, thereby expediting their recovery. Individual treatment sessions are also good as maintenance sessions for clients who require top-up treatments perhaps twice a month, once a month or even once every few months. Such treatments help people keep on top of habitual strain patterns from work, congenital conditions or structural deviations in the body.

Advantages of an Individual Treatment Approach

- Good for an introduction to MFR
- Suits the needs of clients with work and family commitments
- Suits the needs of clients with financial constraints
- Gives clients time to work with their responses to each session
- Gives clients time to work with home programmes
- Good for maintenance programmes
- Good for the client to receive therapy on a one-to-one basis
- Good for therapists with busy schedules (some treatment is better than none)

Disadvantages of an Individual Treatment Approach

- The client may require more therapy than one individual session can offer.
- The treatments may not be regular enough to break habitual holding patterns.

- The client may build up repetitive strain patterns between sessions from work, sport, stress and strain.
- The client may experience only short-term or limited relief and may become despondent and lose faith in the therapy and the ability of the therapist to help.
- The client may forget information about the home programme if treatments are too far apart.

CLIENT TALK

If you have been offering only one-hour sessions, consider offering two hours at a time, or ask the client to commit initially to twice a week to give you time to access the system. Some clients are so bound down that they need more time to feel what is happening and to respond to the therapy.

Intensive Treatment Approaches

Intensive treatments are another fantastic way to immerse the client in the therapy. They provide dramatic results, break habitual holding patterns and release the straitjacket effect on the fascial network. In intensive programmes clients attend therapy for two to three hours per day over four or five days. This can continue over two or three weeks.

An intensive programme allows the therapist not only to perform MFR on a more regular basis but also to provide a relaxation programme that can help the client tune in to the body. A home programme involving therapeutic stretching may be included in an intensive programme, and the therapist may explore with the client what everyday activities may be exacerbating the pain, including helping with ergonomics (the therapeutic design of the working environment) if necessary.

Because intensive programmes occur away from home, clients are placed in new environments, allowing them to focus on themselves and not on their work or other stressors in their lives. They have time to quiet down, rest and relax, which imparts benefits.

CLIENT TALK

If clients are travelling a distance for any MFR treatment, particularly an intensive one, I always recommend that they get someone to drive them or take public transport. They might consider spending an extra day after the treatment before driving home, because long drives can be quite stressful.

Following an intensive therapy treatment, particularly if it has involved a trip away from home, clients can benefit from continuing treatment with a local MFR therapist or a therapist in another modality. They should also plan to make any changes necessary to facilitate their care and not just go back to the stressful environment that contributed to their symptoms.

Intensive programmes can be carried out by one therapist over a few hours, a number of therapists in individual treatment successions or two or three therapists working with one client at the same time. The advantage of multiple therapists is that they often see, feel and pick up on different things. Also, they approach the work differently because of their unique connections with the client. Clients can get used to a style of working that, although beneficial, may be enhanced by the additional points of view of other therapists.

Advantages of an Intensive Treatment Approach

- Gives clients time to immerse themselves totally in the therapy
- Gives the therapist time to treat the entire body
- Breaks habitual holding patterns and releases the straitjacket effect on the fascial network
- Gives the therapist time to deal with issues arising from the previous day's treatment
- Provides the time for the client to use a home programme and other relaxation tools (this depends on the therapist's scope of practice)
- Gives clients the opportunity to focus on themselves

Disadvantages of an Intensive Treatment Approach

- Some clients may find intensive programmes cost prohibitive.
- Clients may not be able to commit the time required for an intensive programme.
- Clients may not be able to stay away from home to attend intensive programmes.
- Clients may not be pain free by the end of an intensive treatment programme. Healing is a journey, not an event.

CLIENT TALK

Having attended a few intensive MFR programmes myself, I can testify to their benefits as a client and to the experience they offer as a therapist. Receiving treatment is one of the most rewarding and beneficial learning environments an MFR therapist can experience.

Multi-Therapist Treatment Approaches

In multi-therapist treatment programmes, more than one therapist works with a client at the same time. This can occur in an individual session or an intensive treatment programme.

Multi-therapist treatments benefit clients in a number of ways. They progress immensely because techniques can be performed more effectively. For example, during a longitudinal plane release with the client lying supine, one therapist can apply traction to an arm whilst another applies traction to a leg. The energy and awareness of both client and therapists are enhanced by the energy of an extra pair of hands. Moreover, habitual holding patterns can be treated more effectively when two therapists apply pressure to the strained and restrictive fascial network.

Advantages of a Multi-Therapist Treatment Approach

- More work can be done in a shorter time; twice the amount of therapy occurs in one hour when two therapists work together.
- Therapy progresses when multiple therapists work together to break habitual holding patterns both emotionally and physically.
- More therapists can offer a greater intuition and awareness of the client's responses to the treatment.
- Clients can see and feel the benefits of the work and generally enjoy the experience.

Disadvantages of a Multi-Therapist Treatment Approach

- Some clients don't like the idea of more than one pair of hands working on them.
- Some clients do not feel well enough to cope with more than one therapist at a time.
- Some clients find multi-therapist treatment sessions cost prohibitive.

TIP Regardless of whether a multi-therapist session occurs during an intensive programme or an individual programme, some clients are not willing to move outside the safety of traditional individual treatments (i.e., one therapist for one hour at a time). Some clients also want to see the same therapist all the time. Although MFR can be successful in these circumstances, clients always benefit from more treatment and a different approach and point of view. You can help your clients understand why longer sessions will help and that receiving treatment from a colleague will offer expertise from a different point of view and even a different skill set.

Home Programmes

Home programmes consist of physical exercises; stretches; relaxation exercises; self-care MFR using balls, foam rolls and other tools; or other activities clients do at home between MFR sessions. Home programmes depend on the remit and scope of practice of the therapist. If you are not allowed to, or have not been trained to, offer home programmes, you should refer your client to a therapist who can provide that service. Home programmes do not need to be complicated or difficult. Two or three components is ideal; more than that usually results in the client's becoming confused or forgetting to do the homework.

Some clients are very keen to expedite their return to normal fitness and health and are willing to do what it takes between treatments. Other clients return to the therapy room admitting to have done no homework since the last session. Both types of clients need encouragement; let them know that if they start with a realistic goal of what is achievable on a daily basis, they will see and feel results.

Fascial tone and ultimately fascial health are best addressed in a variety of ways in home programmes, just as in regular treatment. Home programmes can include components such as proprioception, interoception, flexibility, strength, stamina, and static and dynamic movement. Fascia benefits from fluid movement and compression as well as from stretches in various long axes and planes of movement (e.g., pushing against a wall whilst in a long stance and flexed at the hips).

Home stretching programmes need to mirror the fascial work performed in the MFR treatment. Some clients may be used to stretching as part of a regime for sport, a workout at the gym or a yoga or Pilates class, all of which are effective rehabilitation tools. However, fascial rehabilitation requires that tissue be gently elongated, whereas common forms of stretching take a muscle to its end range of movement and apply a few seconds of stretch to create length. A fascial stretching programme is completely different to a regular stretching programme.

You are now familiar with the sensation of the fascia yielding and softening. Home stretching programmes create those same sensations. You need to educate your clients about how to feel for the barrier, restrictions and end-feel of their own fascial matrix. Teach them how to gently hold that lengthening at the barrier, wait for the tissue to soften and yield, and follow it by leaning into the next barrier, following all changes in the tissues.

Forcing the system with repetitive exercises or stretching, building the core or postural training is not always the answer for many clients. There is no point in applying another straitjacket of tension onto the existing dysfunction or strengthening an opposite muscle group; all this does is tighten the imbalanced system even more. MFR restores function and balance, after which any rehabilitation approach will have maximal benefit.

TIP One of my favourite home programmes is to get clients to notice the normal daily activities that may be exacerbating their dysfunction and discomfort. I may ask clients with shoulder, arm and wrist discomfort, for example, to notice whether they drive with an elbow resting on the windowsill of the car and how they sit at a computer. A key exacerbator of neck, shoulder and jaw issues is the sleeping position. Ask clients with these issues to notice whether they always sleep on the same side or with one arm wrapped around the body or above the head under the pillow. Encourage them, as much as they can, to notice how many times a day and night they are in the same chronic holding pattern. Once they realise and notice how much of their daily habits are exacerbating their dysfunction and discomfort, they will be better able to adapt to new patterns.

Home programmes can include the following:

- Performing two or three stretches or exercises daily between treatments
- A focusing exercise on body awareness, perhaps with music, books, or guided meditation

- Noticing any daily activities or sleeping positions that may be exacerbating the pain
- Building an awareness of stress factors that may be influencing the condition
- Attending other therapies as required

TIP Using a self-care programme yourself that includes easy fascial tools and techniques will help you look after yourself and give you more experience, which in turn will help you develop home programmes for your clients. All fascial home programmes and self-care programmes must reflect the MFR treatment performed in the treatment room. You are essentially performing MFR on yourself and teaching the client to do the same. Clients can be encouraged to use the home programme as soon as they feel any tension or discomfort. In this way, they can be more in control of their bodies and feel less controlled by their conditions.

Care must be taken with all of the following techniques, and clients should be supervised performing them before doing them at home. Make sure your clients know that if they experience any pain or discomfort that is not as a result of an MFR technique, they must stop the technique and discuss it with you at the next treatment.

Longitudinal Planes, Arms and Legs

1. If you are doing this for yourself, you can use your own treatment table. Position yourself side lying on your treatment table in the same position that you use with a client to treat the lateral lumbar with a cross-hand release technique.

2. If you don't have access to your treatment table and for directing a client to use this self-care technique, this same position can be done on a bed taking care not to be too close to the edge.

3. Place the uppermost arm above the head, resting on a pillow or on the side of the head, and the uppermost leg outstretched and slightly behind and off the treatment table or the bed.

4. Make sure your back is always comfortable during this technique.

5. Close your eyes and focus on your body, allowing it to soften.

6. Let go of all of the tension in your body.

7. As your body softens, allow it to move and lengthen into its next barrier and end-feel. Keep noticing where your body softens, maintaining a very subtle lengthening as it changes.

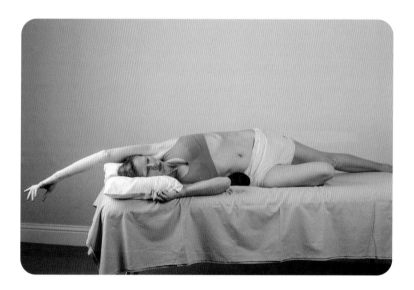

Lying on the Foam Roll

Foam rolls are very popular rehabilitation tools that can be purchased from therapy centres and some sport and fitness outlets, and on the internet. They are long cylinders of dense polystyrene and can be used for stretching and core stability. Foam rolls are excellent for applying and assisting fascial stretching. Many therapists use them daily to compensate for the positions they stand in at their treatment tables. Because therapists tend to stand in a flexed position, the foam roll helps them stretch back into a more neutral position.

Foam rolls can be used in a number of ways, but the application must always be the same. Many people power through movements on foam rolls, but that is not what you want to do with MFR. When using a foam roll, always apply the same principle as with all MFR techniques. Be slow and patient and follow the tissue as it changes. The body must also be as soft as possible lying over or on the foam roll with the exception of the parts that are supporting you.

1. Place the foam roll on the floor. Sit at one end with your knees bent, and very slowly roll backwards onto it so that your spine and head are supported.

2. Keep your feet and knees where they need to be to offer you support.

3. Place your arms down by your sides with your palms facing the ceiling.

4. Close your eyes and focus on your body softening.

5. After a few minutes you will feel your back softening, shoulders widening and chest relaxing.

6. You can easily spend 10 to 15 minutes on a foam roll; however, the emphasis is not on the time spent but the sensations felt.

7. Eventually, as your body softens, move both your arms up higher above your head as if following the numbers on a clock.

8. Wait at each number for your body to soften to maximise the elongation of the tissue.

9. Notice whether your shoulders feel equal and encourage them to soften and balance.

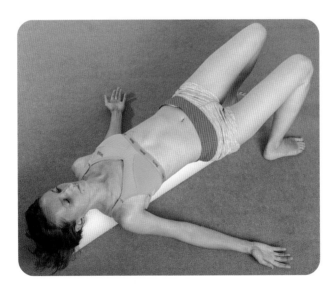

Legs on the Foam Roll

You can also use a foam roll on your back, arms, torso, buttocks and hips.

1. Lie over the foam roll with it under your anterior thighs.
2. Support yourself on your elbows with a pillow or bolster under your abdomen, if required, to support your back.
3. Relax and soften your body over the foam roll, making sure your legs and buttocks are relaxed.
4. Using your elbows, slowly move yourself up or down (top to toe) on the foam roll until you find tissue that feels hot, hard or tender.
5. Soften and wait there until the tissue yields and softens, then roll yourself again until you feel the next restricted and tight area and perform the same approach.
6. This process may take 20 minutes if your legs are really tight, but the emphasis is doing it slowly and diligently in the most relaxed manner to obtain the best results.

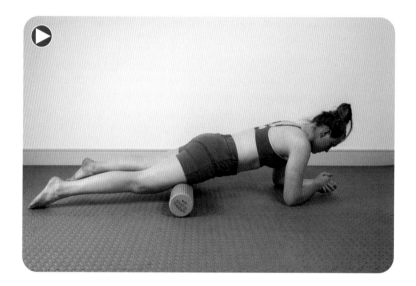

TIP I use the foam roll for self-care whilst lying on my treatment table with my arms over the sides; the edges of the treatment table offer a greater stretch. I also perform cross-hand release techniques and arm pulls on clients when they are on the foam roll, both on the floor and on the treatment table, with the foam roll supported by pillows to enhance the treatment.

Therapy Balls for the Legs and Hips

Therapy balls are plastic balls about 7 to 10 centimetres (3–4 in.) in diameter. They can be smooth or have spikes or knobbles and can be bought from therapy supply shops or on the internet; some children's balls may also work well. Some therapy balls can be inflated and deflated as necessary with a bicycle pump. Working fascially with therapy balls is the same process as working with foam rolls, and they can be used as alternatives to foam rolls at any time.

Therapy balls have become an increasingly popular fascial tool in recent years and are also easy to carry in a suitcase to be used when the client is away on long trips. Consider having a few types of self-care tools available for clients to borrow or try out to see if they like them. At least be prepared to direct clients to places where they can buy the tools you recommend.

1. On the floor, place the ball under one buttock with the same-side leg out-stretched; the opposite leg is flexed at the knee and hip.
2. Support yourself with your arms and flexed leg.
3. Soften down on the ball and gently roll around on your buttock until you find a tender area.
4. Sink down further and wait for the tissue to change.
5. This technique can also be performed side lying to treat the tissue around the head of the greater trochanter, or against a wall with your knees bent and using your legs to lean back into the ball.

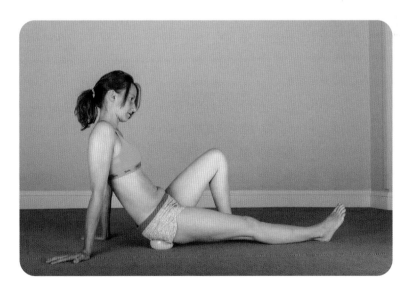

Therapy Ball for the Anterior Hip

1. Place the ball approximately 2 centimetres (0.8 in.) from the anterior superior iliac spine (ASIS) in towards the tummy button and then approximately 2 centimetres (0.8 in.) down towards the inguinal area (crease at the anterior hip).

2. Here you will find your hip flexor muscle (iliopsoas) and usually tight, restricted tissue.

3. Lie on the floor supported on your elbows with the same-side leg stretched and the ball at your anterior hip.

4. Bend your other leg at the knee and the hip, and externally rotate it out to the side.

5. Keep your hips level and allow your buttocks, legs and back to soften and slowly sink down onto the ball.

6. Roll gently to find the area of increased tension.

7. Wait for the tissue to soften.

8. Once you feel the tissues stretch, you can enhance the technique by slowly flexing the knee of your straight leg.

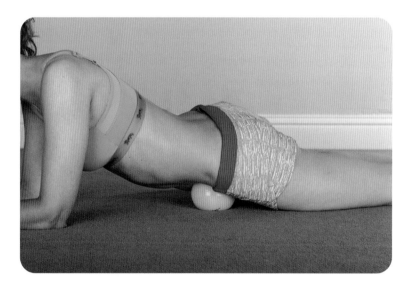

CLIENT TALK

People who have had low back injuries should take special care during this technique. People who are pregnant or those who are trying to become pregnant must not do abdominal work.

Therapy Ball for the Neck and Shoulders

1. Leaning up against a wall, bend your knees and lean your body back into the ball.
2. Side bend, forward bend or rotate your neck to increase the stretch.
3. Allow your shoulders to soften.
4. Sink back onto the ball and slowly roll until you find an area of increased tension, then wait for a feeling of tissue yielding and softening.
5. To use the ball on the upper shoulder area, you will need to bend your knees to increase the backward angle to reach this area.
6. Smaller soft rubber balls can be used to treat your hands and feet by leaning into the ball on the floor or on a firm surface.

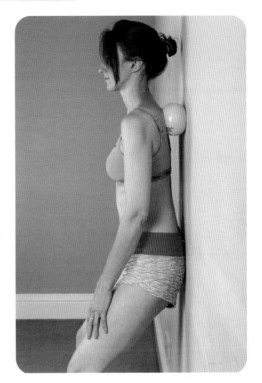

CLIENT TALK

Many therapists now do self-myofascial release (SMFR) therapy. In these sessions, which can be completed over a video call or face to face, the therapist teaches the client how to use therapy tools to help themselves. Online SMFR therapy classes, taught by a trained therapist, are also available. SMFR therapy primarily uses balls and foam rolls but many advanced classes also address fascial stretching and the use of other tools such as myofascial peanut rollers specifically designed for the back or other areas with tension.

Closing Remarks

Regardless of whether you are performing an individual, intensive or multi-therapist session, always take the needs of the client into consideration. Never force clients to do things they are not ready to do.

Some clients are quite happy to mix intensive and individual treatments by attending regular individual therapy and at intermittent intervals attending an intensive. Some clients prefer to have individual sessions first before committing to an intensive, whereas others prefer the opposite. All are equally acceptable and can provide lasting results.

Home and self-care programmes can help you cope with the demands of a busy clinic and experience fascial work first hand. You can then take your increased body awareness to your clients through treatments and home care programmes.

Quick Questions

1. What is the difference between an intensive treatment programme and a multi-therapist treatment programme?
2. Should you supervise clients performing home programme components before they attempt them at home?
3. What are the advantages of an intensive treatment programme?
4. Should pregnant people perform home programmes on the abdominal area?
5. Will self-care programmes increase your own body awareness?

Chapter 1

1. Muscles have an insertion and an origin. Fascia is completely continuous; therefore, techniques can ultimately influence the entire matrix. Fascia also resists force that is applied too quickly and with too much pressure. Less is more with fascia.
2. Bound water is a colloidal liquid crystal that is highly viscoelastic and forms in the presence of a hydrophilic tissue—in this case, the collagen protein.
3. Adipose or fat tissue
4. Approximately 90 to 120 seconds
5. Collagen, elastin and the ground substance

Chapter 2

1. Clients often know more about their conditions than you do and thus can offer valuable insight to help you in the treatment.
2. The thickness of a wallet or phone will push the pelvis upwards, forwards or backwards, creating a muscular holding pattern and causing an imbalance and subsequent dysfunction.
3. Anterior, posterior, right and left lateral and transverse view down the back of the client's body
4. Yes, always
5. The jawbone

Chapter 3

1. The answer to this question depends on your scope of practice. If you already work with pregnant people, then yes, you can use MFR if you are insured to do so. Some organisations and professional associations ask that you attend a pregnancy massage course first and obtain the relevant insurance.
2. With local contraindications, no therapy should be performed on the affected body part. With global contraindications, the client should not receive MFR at all.
3. Keep your back straight and do not bend over the treatment table when performing MFR.

4. Engaging the client in the process by using effective dialoguing and descriptions of the treatment will help the client understand the therapy and its responses and effects. This will enhance the results of the treatment.

5. For the process of MFR to work, the client needs to be focused, aware of the response to treatment and relaxed. This cannot happen when both client and therapist are not concentrating on the work.

Chapter 4

1. *Mobility* means 'tissue movement' or how well the tissues move.

2. The end-feel is where the tissue gliding ends as a result of a restriction or a limitation of the end of range of the tissues.

3. The anterior superior iliac spines

4. Myofascial rebounding

5. Yes. It is best to use both methods to obtain a more precise assessment of the tissues.

Chapter 5

1. No, these products will cause your hands to slip on the skin, and you will not be able to engage the tissues below.

2. Longitudinal plane releases

3. Analytical questions may make clients try to work out and judge what they are feeling. Encourage them to avoid the thinking process and to feel what is happening instead.

4. Fascia is aligned predominantly top to toe.

5. Three to five minutes, sometimes longer depending on the client

Chapter 6

1. No. MFR is a whole-body approach and, as such, is based on the principle of treating the entire system to promote balance and function.

2. Care must be taken in client positioning for the cross-hand release of the lateral lumbar. A small pillow must be placed beneath the client's waist to keep the spine neutral. Make sure the client is comfortable at all times during the technique, and help the client bring the arm and leg on the side you are working on back to neutral after completing the technique.

3. No. Any MFR on the abdominal area is contraindicated at all stages of pregnancy.

4. The anterior superior iliac spine (ASIS)

5. No. We never use massage oil or lotion to perform MFR.

Chapter 7

1. Supine, prone and side lying
2. A small pillow, bolster or rolled-up towel must be placed to keep the lumbar spine in the low back area neutral.
3. You must avoid squeezing or holding too tight. Always hold the lower arm in a gentle but secure way.
4. Traction, external rotation and abduction
5. Probably not. You should take care to stay within the client's range of movement, which will differ from client to client.

Chapter 8

1. No, your hands stay side by side.
2. Yes
3. Yes
4. Prone and supine
5. Traction techniques, usually longitudinal plane release techniques (arm and leg pulls)

Chapter 9

1. Yes, always look for red flare or a vasomotor response during or after all MFR techniques.
2. The pelvic floor, respiratory diaphragm, thoracic inlet and cranial base
3. Your thumbs must always be pointing towards the client's head, and you should obtain permission to place your hands skin on skin in this area. Alternatives are including a layer of clothing or allowing the client to place their own hand on the skin over the suprapubic area.
4. Yes, they can also be performed with the client seated or standing.
5. Three to five minutes, sometimes more

Chapter 10

1. Six weeks after surgery or injury
2. Skin rolling
3. Yes, skin rolling is good for treating possible adhesions from abdominal surgery or injury.
4. Yes, position of ease techniques compress the tissue back towards the restriction.
5. A keloid scar

Chapter 11

1. They are pin and stretch, level techniques and direct MFR.
2. Myofascial mobilisations are normally performed in longitudinal and transverse directions.
3. The proximal phalanges are the parts of your fingers closest to the bones of your hand.
4. We are treating the gastrocnemius and the soleus muscles in the calf technique.
5. No, you shouldn't do the iliopsoas myofascial mobilisation technique on a person who is pregnant or is trying to become pregnant.

Chapter 12

1. The art of MFR is following what you feel. You can therefore integrate what you feel you need to do, as well as follow the client's body as you perceive the tissue changes, to obtain the best result for your client. There are no recipes or protocols in MFR.
2. The position that offers the least resistance
3. Yes, despite skin rolling being part of an assessment for restrictions, it can still be integrated as a technique with all other MFR techniques.
4. By receiving treatment and attending hands-on workshops
5. Three to five minutes

Chapter 13

1. An intensive programme is a series of treatments over days and sometimes weeks; a multi-therapist programme can be an individual session with two or more therapists.
2. Yes, you need to ensure that clients can perform home programme components safely and correctly.
3. An intensive treatment programme allows clients to completely immerse themselves in the therapy to create change. It also breaks the bracing and holding patterns that affect health and gives the therapist time to treat the entire body and address issues that arise from the previous day's session before further compensatory patterns can occur.
4. No, abdominal work should be avoided for the duration of the pregnancy.
5. Yes, receiving any kind of MFR therapy will help you become more aware and develop your kinaesthetic touch whilst also keeping your body in good shape to prevent injury.

References

Chapter 1

Barnes, J.F. 1990. Myofascial release: The search for excellence—A comprehensive evaluatory and treatment approach. Paoli/Malvern, PA: Rehabilitation Services.

Bhowmick, S., Singh, A., Flavell, R.A., Clark, R.B., O'Rourke, J., and Cone, R.E. 2009. The sympathetic nervous system modulates CD4+FoxP3+ regulatory T cells via a TGF-beta-dependent mechanism. *Journal of Leukocyte Biology* 86 (6): 1275–1283.

Chaitow, L., and DeLany, J. 2008. *The upper body*. Vol. 1 of *Clinical application of neuromuscular techniques*. 2nd edition. Philadelphia: Churchill Livingstone.

Chaitow, L. 2017. What's in a name: Myofascial release or myofascial induction? *Journal of Bodywork and Movement Therapies* 21(4): 749–751. https://doi:10.1016/j.jbmt.2017.09.008

Chaitow, L., 2018. *Fascial Dysfunction. Manual therapy approaches*. 2nd edition. Edinburgh: Handspring.

Craig, A.D. 2003. Interoception: The sense of the physiological condition of the body. *Current Opinion in Neurobiology* 13 (4): 500–505. https://doi.org/10.1016/S0959-4388(03)00090-4.

Fede, C., Albertin, G., Petrelli, L., Sfriso, M.M., Biz, C., De Caro, R., and Stecco, C. 2016. Hormone receptor expression in human fascial tissue. *European Journal of Histochemistry* 60 (4): 224–229. https://doi.org/10.4081/ejh.2016.2710.

Findley, T., Chaudhry, H., and Dhar, S. 2015. Transmission of muscle force to fascia during exercise. *Journal of Bodywork and Movement Therapies* 19 (1): 119–123. https://doi.org/10.1016/j.jbmt.2014.08.010.

Huijing, P.A. 2007. Epimuscular myofascial force transmission between antagonistic and synergistic muscles can explain movement limitation in spastic paresis. *Journal of Electromyography and Kinesiology* 17 (6): 708–724. https://doi.org/10.1016/j.jelekin.2007.02.003.

Huijing, P.A., and Langevin, H.M. 2009. Communicating about fascia: History, pitfalls, and recommendations. *International Journal of Therapeutic Massage and Bodywork* 2 (4): 3–8.

Huijing, P.A., Maas, H., and Baan, G.C. 2003. Compartmental fasciotomy and isolating a muscle from neighboring muscles interfere with myofascial force transmission within the rat anterior crural compartment. *Journal of Morphology* 256 (3): 306–321. https://doi.org/10.1002/jmor.10097.

Juhan, D. 2003. *Job's body: A handbook for bodywork*. 3rd edition. Barrytown, NY: Station Hill of Barrytown.

Katake, K. 1961. The strength for tension and bursting of human fascia. *Journal of Kyoto Prefectural University of Medicine* 69: 484–488.

Langevin, H.M. 2006. Connective tissue: A body-wide signalling network? *Medical Hypotheses* 66 (6): 1074–1077.

Meltzer, K.R., Cao, T.V., Schad, J.F., King, H., Stoll, S.T., and Standley, P.R. 2010. In vitro modeling of repetitive motion injury and myofascial release. *Journal of Bodywork and Movement Therapies* 14 (2): 162–171.

Menon, R.G., Oswald, S.F., Raghavan, P., Regatte, R.R., and Stecco, A. 2020. $T_{1\rho}$-mapping for musculoskeletal pain diagnosis: Case series of variation of water bound glycosaminoglycans quantification before and after Fascial Manipulation® in subjects with elbow pain. *International*

Journal of Environmental Research and Public Health 17 (3): 1–10. https://doi.org/10.3390/ijerph17030708.

Moseley, G.L., Zalucki, N.M., and Wiech, K. 2008. Tactile discrimination, but not tactile stimulation alone, reduces chronic limb pain. *Pain* 137 (3): 600–608.

Pischinger, A. 2007. *The extracellular matrix and ground regulations: Basis for a holistic biological medicine.* Berkeley, CA: North Atlantic Books.

Pollack, G.H. 2013. *The fourth phase of water: Beyond solid, liquid, and vapor.* Seattle: Ebner and Sons.

Schleip, R. 2017. Fascia as a sensory organ. In T. Liem, P. Tozzi, & A. Chila (Eds.), *Fascia in the osteopathic field.* Edinburgh: Handspring Publishing.

Schleip, Robert. 2021. Innervation of the Fascia. In D. Lesondak & A.M. Akey (Eds.), *Fascia, function and medical applications.* Boca Raton, FL: Taylor & Francis Group LLC.

Schleip, Robert, Findley, T.W., Chaitow, L., & Huijing, P. 2012. Introduction. In R. Schleip, T.W. Findley, L. Chaitow, & P. Huijing (Eds.), *Fascia: The tensional network of the human body.* Philadelphia: Churchill Livingstone.

Selye, H. 1955. Stress and disease. *Science* 122 (3171): 625–631.

Standley, P., and Metzer, K. 2008. In vitro modeling of repetitive motion strain and manual medicine treatments: Potential roles for pro- and anti-inflammatory cytokines. *Journal of Bodywork and Movement Therapies* 12(3) 201–203. https://doi.org/10.1016/j.jbmt.2008.05.006.

Stecco, C., Fede, C., Macchi, V., Porzionato, A., Petrelli, L., Biz, C., Stern, R., and de Caro, R. 2018. The fasciacytes: A new cell devoted to fascial gliding regulation. *Clinical Anatomy* 31 (5): 667–676. https://doi.org/10.1002/ca.23072.

Stecco, C., and Schleip, R. 2016. A fascia and the fascial system. *Journal of Bodywork and Movement Therapies* 20 (1): 139–140. https://doi.org/10.1016/j.jbmt.2015.11.012.

Stecco, C., Stern, R., Porzionato, A., MacChi, V., Masiero, S., Stecco, A., and de Caro, R. 2011. Hyaluronan within fascia in the etiology of myofascial pain. *Surgical and Radiologic Anatomy* 33 (10): 891–896. https://doi.org/10.1007/s00276-011-0876-9.

Tesarz, J., Hoheisel, U., Wiedenhöfer, B., and Mense, S. 2011. Sensory innervation of the thoracolumbar fascia in rats and humans. *Neuroscience* 194 (October 2011): 302–308. https://doi.org/10.1016/j.neuroscience.2011.07.066.

Chapter 4

Chaitow, L. 2010. *Palpation and assessment skills: Assessment through touch*, 3rd edition. Philadelphia: Churchill Livingstone.

Page, P., Frank, C., and Lardner, R. 2010. *Assessment and treatment of muscle imbalances: The Janda approach.* Champaign, IL: Human Kinetics.

Chapter 5

Bove, G.M., Chapelle, S.L., Hanlon, K.E., Diamond, M.P., and Mokler, D.J. 2017. Attenuation of postoperative adhesions using a modeled manual therapy. *PLoS ONE* 12 (6): 1–18. https://doi.org/10.1371/journal.pone.0178407.

Assessments

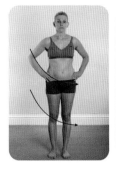

Postural   p. 44

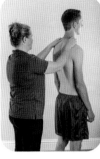

Palpatory   p. 69

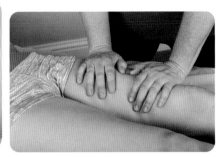

Tissue Mobility and Motility   p. 75

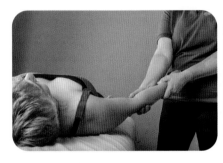

Traction and Compression   p. 79

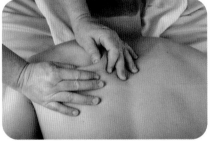

Skin Rolling   p. 82

Myofascial Releases
Cross-Hand Releases

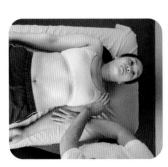

Arm   p. 112

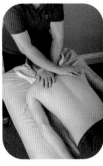

Torso   p. 118

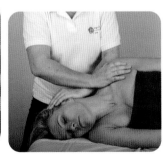

Head and Neck   p. 121

> continued

Myofascial Releases   *>continued*
Longitudinal Plane Releases

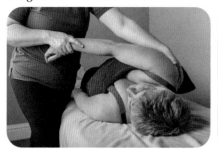

Supine Pulls   p. 127

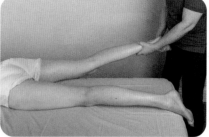

Prone Pulls   p. 132

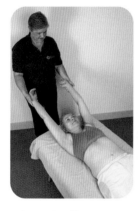

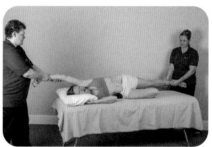

Bilateral Pulls   p. 133   *Oppositional and Side-Lying Pulls*   p. 136

Compression Releases

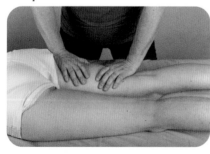

Soft Tissue Compression   p. 144

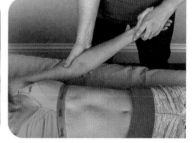

Joint Compression   p. 146

Transverse Plane Releases

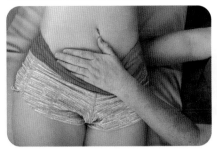

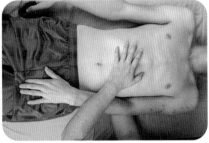

Pelvic Floor   p. 150   *Respiratory Diaphragm*   p. 151

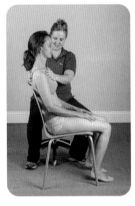

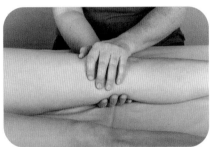

Thoracic Inlet   p. 153   *At Joints*   p. 154

Scar Tissue

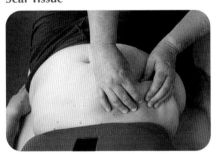

Skin Rolling   p. 160

> *continued*

Myofascial Releases   *>continued*
Direct Scar Tissue Release

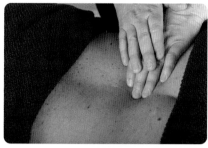

Mobilisation   p. 169

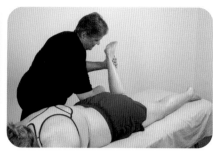

Piriformis   p. 174

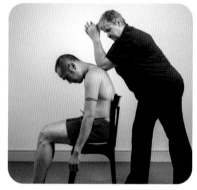

Erector Spinae Muscle   p. 187

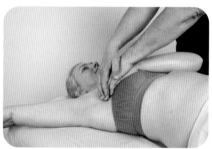

Pectoralis Muscle   p. 188

Other Myofascial Techniques

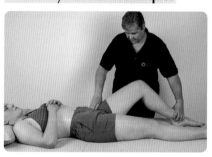

Psoas and Iliacus   p. 191

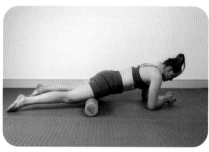

Home Programmes   p. 218

About the Author

Ruth Duncan, BSc (Hons), MSMTO, is an advanced myofascial release therapist, proprietor, instructor, guest lecturer, speaker, national committee member and writer with extensive training in a variety of approaches. She completed her advanced postgraduate training in 2004 with John F. Barnes (the world's leading authority on myofascial release) and has assisted with his seminars in the United States.

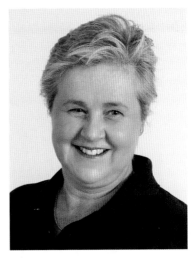

Courtesy of Joyce Martin Photography.

Duncan also has explored other direct and nondirect fascial approaches, including Thomas Myers' anatomy trains and myofascial meridians, Erik Dalton's myoskeletal alignment techniques and Jean-Pierre Barral's visceral manipulation. She has studied with experts on myriad topics to learn more about human anatomy, function and dysfunction, and the emotional aspects of chronic pain and healing.

Duncan graduated with honours as a clinical massage therapist from the Humanities Center School of Massage (now the Cortiva Institute) in Florida, United States. She has a diploma in sports therapy from the Society of Sports Therapists and a diploma in sports and remedial massage from the Institute of Sport and Remedial Massage. She also has a BSc in health sciences from The Open University and a PGCert in pain science and theory from the University of South Australia. She has been teaching myofascial release in the United Kingdom and internationally for over 15 years.

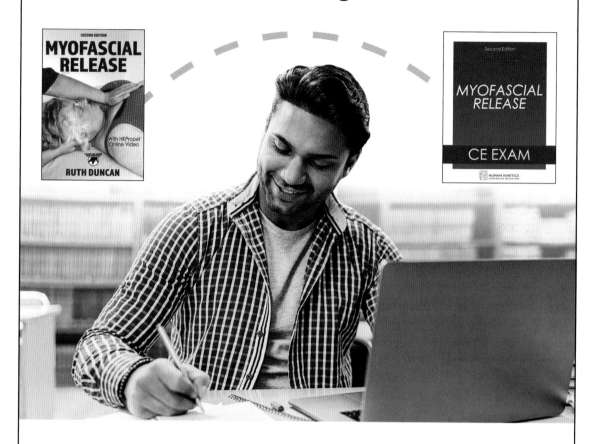
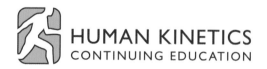